DANCE
MEDICINE

Head to Toe

A Dancer's Guide to Health

DANCE
MEDICINE

Head to Toe

A Dancer's Guide to Health

JUDITH R. PETERSON, MD

ILLUSTRATIONS BY
KATHLEEN ROWLAND

PRINCETON BOOK COMPANY, PUBLISHERS

NOTICE AND DISCLAIMER

This book is intended as a reference only.

This information is not intended to be nor should be used as a substitute for direct, personal, professional medical care and diagnosis. The information contained within is not intended to provide specific physical or mental health advice for any individual and should not be relied upon in that regard. Prior to engaging in the exercises in this book, you should consult with your personal physician. If you suspect that you have a medical problem or are experiencing any health issues, it is recommended that you seek competent medical care and to consult with your personal physician immediately.

Copyright © 2011 by Judith R. Peterson
All rights reserved

Library of Congress Cataloging-in-Publication Data
Peterson, Judith R.
  Dance medicine, head to toe : a dancer's guide to health / Judith R. Peterson ; illustrations by Kathleen Rowland.

    p. : ill. ; cm.

  Includes bibliographical references and index.
  ISBN: 978-0-87127-352-9 (hardcover)
  ISBN: 978-0-87127-353-6 (pbk.)

    1. Dancers--Health and hygiene. 2. Dancing injuries--Prevention. 3. Dancers--Nutrition. 4. Dance--Health aspects. 5. Dance--Physiological aspects. I. Rowland, Kathleen. II. Title.

RC1220.D35 P48 2011
613.62

Princeton Book Company, Publishers
614 Route 130
Hightstown, NJ 08520-0831

Design and composition by High Tide Design

Contents

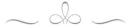

Acknowledgements

Thank you to my fabulous illustrator, Kathleen Rowland, who brought this text to life. Thank you to Pennsylvania Ballet for their support over the years and the use of the beautiful dance photography throughout this book. In particular, at Pennsylvania Ballet, thank you to Artistic Director Roy Kaiser and his assistant, Michael Sheridan. Thank you to Sandra D'Amelio Racowski at Pennsylvania Ballet for help with many issues over many years. And also at Pennsylvania Ballet, thank you to Marissa Montenegro for help with coordinating photo access and many other minute, yet important, tasks!

Thank you very much to my publisher, Charles Woodford, and the staff of Princeton Book Company, Publishers, for all of their help and encouragement in the creation of this book.

Thank you to Gayeanne Grossman, Julie Green, and Ruth Scott—three extraordinary dance physical therapists with whom I have had the privilege of working on many projects and who each helped with this book. Thank you to Dr. William Morrison and Thomas Jefferson University Hospital (Philadelphia) for the use of the radiographic images in this book. Thank you very much to Anna Gieschen, research librarian, whose efforts were such an enormous help. Thank you to all of the dancers over all of the years for being an ongoing source of inspiration to me.

Thank you to my husband, Michael, and my two daughters, Alison and Lisa. And finally, this book could not have been completed if my cat, Hayden, had not gotten up from the keyboard occasionally, so a big thank you to little Hayden, as well.

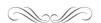

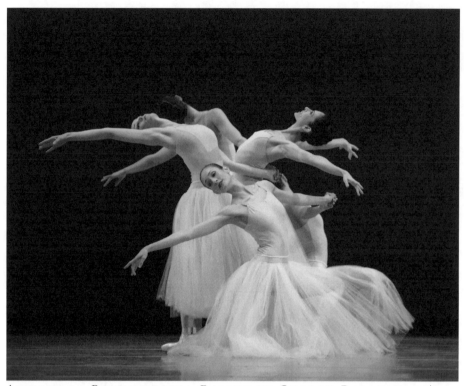

ARTISTS OF PENNSYLVANIA BALLET IN GEORGE BALANCHINE'S
SERENADE. PHOTOGRAPH BY PAUL KOLNIK.

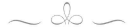

Introduction

This is a book about dancers' health. It is meant to help you understand your health and how some of the demands of dance may affect your health. I hope that with this focus on health, you can be the dancer who is pro-active about your health and wellness. Becoming healthy and remaining healthy is a lifetime's work! You cannot do it by yourself. But I sincerely hope that this book helps you start toward a lifetime of dance that is healthy for you!

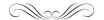

1 The Beginning

Fostering Dancers' Mental Health

DANCE IS GREAT FOR YOU. THIS IS PROBABLY THE MOST IMPORTANT SENTENCE ABOUT DANCE ANYONE CAN SAY AND THAT IS WHY IT IS THE FIRST SENTENCE OF THIS BOOK. THE EXERCISE OF DANCE HELPS BUILD YOUR MUSCLES AND KEEPS YOUR BONES STRONG. DANCE IS BEAUTIFUL AND INSPIRING. DANCE PROMOTES MENTAL AND PHYSICAL DISCIPLINE. DANCE WILL FOREVER CHANGE YOUR CONCEPTS OF RHYTHM AND MUSICALITY.

BUT—dancers also know that the world of dance is a demanding one. Dancers do the grinding and repetitive work that makes movement appear effortless. This endless repetition in the pursuit of perfection and grace can take a toll on the dancer's body and psyche. Real mental and physical distress can be the consequence. More than half of all dancers eventually will become injured, and some articles even comment on nearly universal injury rates—that up to 90% of dancers get injured (US Department of Labor, Bureau of Labor Statistics). Injuries in dancers are often from overuse or muscular imbalances. Problems in dance technique may go uncorrected and lead to problems and pain. These injuries can cause the end of an aspiring and talented dancer's career. Injury is one commonly cited reason that dancers discontinue training and performance.

SELF-CRITICISM AND DANCE

Dance is one of the few athletic activities that requires long periods of practice staring into a mirror and self-criticizing. It is difficult to do this for hours on end. In the studio, the dancers look at themselves, dancers look at each other, the teacher looks at the dancers…and on and on. Dancers criticize themselves. They may criticize each other. The teacher paces up and down the lines of the dancers and frowns or nods. Dancers may wonder, "What will the teacher think? Am I really the worst dancer in this class? Am I the slowest to learn this choreography?"

It is hard for most people to be working under this type of constant scrutiny, and yet this is the daily life of the dancer. And of course, the way that we become better dancers is through this at-times-brutal self-criticism and the advice of our classmates and teachers. Valerie Grieg says, "We learn to dance by dancing" (Grieg 1994, xiii). It is very important to remember this to stay mentally strong and positive despite criticism. Ballet is as demanding as football, basketball, and ice hockey in the mental dedication required and is as physically demanding as many strenuous sports (Maffulli, 162). So to dance you need to strengthen yourself mentally as well as physically.

When you are in class, remember that class really is about this mental and physical strengthening process. Be kind to yourself as you criticize how you are doing in class! If you misstep, it is just that—a misstep, not a complete condemnation of all your dance achievements. It is called dance *class* because it is the time for your body and mind to coordinate and learn the programs and movements prior to your time on stage.

The mind/body connection is a real one. Your brain constantly communicates with your muscles to get the movements of the dance to flow. If you become overwhelmed by the classroom or the teacher, your brain will make your muscles become tense — and a tense dancer is not a dancer performing to his or her best abilities.

Body Image Issues and Dance

Dancers look thinner than most people. There are probably a variety of reasons why dance emphasizes that slender look. The mirrors, the teacher, the other students, the dancer's own self-image, and some choreographers' preferences influence this look. Clothing that shows every skin dimple, and training that melts away body fat also contribute. The weigh-in ritual that persists at some dance academies is likely a weight-controlling factor at those institutions, as well.

Is that the way it is, then? Are an eating disorder and psychological distress the inevitable destiny of the dancer? The answer is no! Rachel Bachner-Melman and her colleagues (Bachner-Melman et al. 2006) studied the psychological distress of aesthetic athletes, those involved in a sport in which the appearance of the athlete could influence the outcome of a competition. In the study, the aesthetic athletes were predominately dancers, but the group included gymnasts, synchronized swimmers, and athletes in other sports. Non-aesthetic sports are those like basketball in which the only way to win points is to get the ball through the basketball hoop; whether the ball gets in the hoop is not affected by the look of the athlete. The non-aesthetic athletes in the study participated in sports such as running and basketball.

In the study, the aesthetic athletes, generally speaking, had matched psychological profiles with the non-athletic control group. There was no difference in their perfectionist tendencies or self-esteem. A greater number of women with eating disorders, however, were found in the aesthetic athletes. It is thought that perhaps the environmental pressures of dance lead to the exaggerated emphasis on thinness in certain of these athletes as compared to the control group.

Stress and Injury

Stress makes you edgy, tight, and mentally scattered. Your heart rate goes up; your concentration goes down. The American College of Sports Medicine (2006) has issued a consensus statement about stress and its impact on athletes. Stress in athletes causes injury. Dancers need to be aware of this as they have unique kinds of stress.

Do any of the following symptoms sound like you? Feeling overwhelmed; trouble sleeping; using alcohol or pills or over the counter substances to wind up, chill out, or calm down enough to get through your day? Can't perform well in public, snap out at friends and family? Can't eat, can't stop eating? Endless self-doubt, nonstop self-criticism? Endless fatigue, tired all the time, wired all the time? All of the preceding symptoms and complaints can be signs of stress or other psychological issues that have a negative effect on your health generally and your risk of injury specifically.

How can I regain some control over my stress?

Eric Franklin (1996) has written extensively on the role of thought and imagery as helpful aids to decreasing bodily stress and improving performance. As Franklin says, "Tension is not a good state of readiness because it exhausts the muscles…" (Franklin 1996, 282). He is pointing out the simple reality that if you are already contracted from tension throughout your body it is going to be pretty tough to perform a relaxed and purposeful movement.

There are some exercises that can help you eliminate this tension from your muscles. Franklin suggests visualization exercises such as imagining the central axis of the body as one straight pole and allowing the "blankets" that form the outer aspect of the body to collapse softly to the center. Another great visualization exercise from Franklin to help with tension is to imagine your outer body as a group of clouds that float and, as you move, move with you (Franklin 1996, 283). Or your body can be a string that hangs down from the top of your head, easing you into perfect alignment (Franklin 1996, 282).

What are relaxation exercises? How do I meditate?

Relaxation techniques are used as a way to decrease muscle tension and mental tension. Relaxation exercises, which can be done in a variety of ways, help

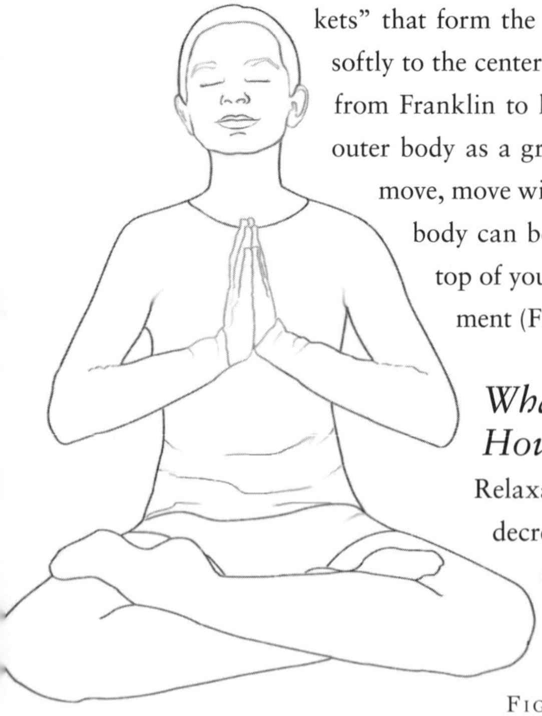

FIG 1-1: DANCER SITTING IN MEDITATION

decrease stress and promote better overall health. One technique uses visualization to help promote this decrease in muscle tightness. Visualization also will help your mental focus if you practice the techniques regularly. For example, imagine that your head is a balloon. Slowly let your head rise up. You will feel your neck and shoulders beginning to relax and yield their tension. You are using the visualization process to retrain the muscles that are holding tension.

Meditation exercises can be very helpful, too. "Walking meditation" is a terrific way to start being mindful of your body and how you move through space. Instead of focusing on the destination, whether there is a Starbucks™ on the way, if you left your leotard at the dance studio, etc., etc., you focus on the journey and the experience of the walk. You walk for twenty minutes or so without a destination, focusing on the grace of your steps as you follow a peaceful path. With each step, be aware of the lifting and placement of your foot. This contemplative walking can be described as "walking meditation."

You do not have to walk to meditate. You can sit and meditate (Fig. 1-1). And you can start right now.

How right now? In the book *8 Minute Meditation*, Victor Davich (2004) talks about simply sitting down and beginning to meditate. In the "minute meditation," you sit straight up, close your eyes, take a deep breath, and then start breathing in a natural way. Feel where your breath seems to concentrate itself. Is it in your diaphragm? Is it in your nose? There is no wrong answer! Simply note where your breathing cycle concentrates. Focus on your breathing for a cycle of five breaths.

Just as we walked contemplatively, thinking about our steps, we have now practiced breathing contemplatively, thinking about each breath. You have focused on the present moment and used body awareness to promote both concentration and relaxation. This simple, sitting, breathing exercise is a form of meditation. You have better awareness of your body without exerting force to control your body. This type of stress reduction exercise can help make you a more focused, yet more relaxed, dancer (Davich 2004, 13).

There are many additional techniques other than meditation or visual imagery that may help with stress. The following list from the American College of Sports Medicine (2004), suggests some additional techniques to help you cope with stress: cognitive-based techniques; somatic-based techniques; cognitive-behavioral techniques; thought stopping; slow, deep, or centered breathing; goal setting; thought replacement and imagery; stress management training; positive self talk; biofeedback training; and progressive muscle relaxation.

If you have stress that is interfering with your health, try stress reduction techniques and, if necessary, get yourself help from a qualified mental health professional.

WHY CAN'T I SLEEP?

Young dancers with sleep issues stumble through days in a fatigued fog and then appear in dance class. The dancer might get the choreography—or not—(because of mental fatigue) and then that dancer stumbles home at night, to again stay up too late, and then repeats this process the next day. Drs. Acebo and Carskadon found that sleep-deprived teenagers and teenagers with irregular sleep patterns have more trouble with day-to-day functioning (Acebo and Carskadon [2002] 2010, 220–221). In addition, lack of sleep may affect the body's ability to fight infection because the lack of sleep may suppress your immune function of your lymph system. Finally, lack of sleep may be a significant factor in traumatic accidents such as car crashes. In fact, 37% of the driving population says they have nodded off for at least a moment or fallen asleep while driving at some time in their life (NHTSA 2002).

This means that sleep deprivation is an enormous public health problem. The United States Navy has been concerned enough about the effects of loss of sleep to formally recommend that the young recruits have a later wake time so they could get a longer period of sleep (Grady 2002).

How do you know if you have a sleep disorder or sleep deprivation issue?

Here are some clues that can help you figure out if you have insomnia or another sleep problem. If you snore, if you have been told you hold your breath when you sleep, if you fall asleep doing homework or watching television, if you sleep-walk, if your legs jump around at night—you could have a sleep issue. If you have trouble getting to sleep, staying asleep, waking up, or if you experience a morning headache, fatigue throughout the day, or trouble concentrating—you could have a sleep disorder. Get yourself checked out!

How can I get better sleep?

There are simple steps you can take to get better sleep. First of all, try not to exercise late at night. A break of a few hours between class and sleep time will be beneficial. Stay away from the gym right before you try to go to sleep. Also, as your body cools down, it is better able to fall asleep. Second, caffeine takes about six hours to break down in your body. So, if you have a large coffee one hour after dinner, you are taking in a whopping 330 mg. of caffeine, which will make it hard for you to sleep! If you can keep your caffeine intake to fewer than 200 mg. of caffeine daily, particularly late at night near your bedtime, you will help yourself get sleep.

Try to think about developing a good sleep routine. Dancers are organized about work and class time. You can think about sleep as an important extension of class time as it provides your body with an opportunity to heal. Choose a certain hour when you will start winding down from the day's activities and putting work and reading materials away. Create a pre-sleep sequence that you try to adhere to most of the time. Finally, the cell phone, the Twitter account, the email, Facebook, television: removing these distractions from the bedroom can be helpful for sleep.

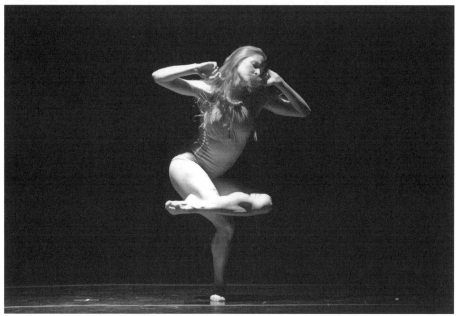

PENNSYLVANIA BALLET COMPANY MEMBER ABIGAIL MENTZER IN ANNABELLE LOPEZ OCHOA'S *REQUIEM FOR A ROSE*. PHOTOGRAPH BY ALEXANDER IZILIAEV.

INJURY AND DANCE

Most dancers will get an injury at some point, and most dancers are also slow to report injuries! There may be fear that the dancer will be cut from the cast list, or worse yet, be told not to dance at all. However, this reluctance to seek treatment is not helpful. Delaying needed care can make it much harder for an injury to heal. In fact, if the dancer is not using his or her body correctly he or she may suffer additional injuries. Yet studies show time and again that dancers frequently delay, delay, delay getting treatment (Krasnow et al. 1994). Pain is your body's way of explaining to you that something is not correct. If you are injured, in pain, or think there may be an issue, get yourself checked.

Four things to know about your mind/body connection

1. Dancers can have high amounts of stress.

2. High amounts of stress can increase your risk of injury.

3. Stress can cause tight muscles, poor sleep, problems concentrating, and burnout...

4. Getting proper amounts of rest and eating a reasonable diet can help minimize the effects of stress and the effects of injury.

Manage your stress! Five techniques that help

There are techniques that help manage stress and you should get in the habit of using them. Here are five simple things you can do:

1. Cross-train and force yourself to do an activity that is different from dance.

2. Find friends who are not involved in dance and find activities that are not focused on dance. Develop a creative space to allow a life that is outside of dance.

3. Get enough sleep.

4. Meditation can be a great way to get control of anxiety and generally calm down. You do not need special equipment and you can call on the meditation techniques when you need them.

5. Staying in good general physical condition can be a terrific help to staying in good general mental condition.

References

Acebo, Christine and Mary Carskadon. (2002) 2010. "Influence of Irregular Sleep Patterns on Waking Behavior." In *Adolescent Sleep Patterns: Biological, Social, and Psychological Influences*, edited by Mary Carskadon, 220–235. Paperbound edition. Cambridge, UK: Cambridge University Press.

American College of Sports Medicine. 2006. "Psychological Issues Related to Injuries in Athletes and the Team Physician: A Consensus Statement." *Medicine and Science in Sport and Exercise* 38 (11): 2030–2034.

Bachner-Melman, Rachel, Ada Zohar, Richard P. Ebstein, Yoel Elizur, and Naama Constantini. 2006. "How Anorexic-like Are the Symptom and Personality Profiles of Aesthetic Athletes?" *Medicine and Science in Sport and Exercise* 38 (4): 2030–2034.

Bodian, Stephan. 2006. *Meditation for Dummies,* 2nd edition. Hoboken, NJ: Wiley.

Bureau of Labor Statistics, US Department of Labor, Occupational Outlook Handbook, 2010-11 Edition, Dancers and Choreographers, on the internet at http: //www.bls.gov/oco/ocos094.htm

Chawla, Jasvinder, MD and Amer Suleman, MD. 2008. "Neurologic Effects of Caffeine." *eMedicine/Neurology*, November 26. http://emedicine.medscape.com/article/1182710-overview.

Davich, Victor. 2004. *8 Minute Meditation: Quiet Your Mind, Change Your Life*. New York: Penguin USA.

Franklin, Eric. 1996. *Dynamic Alignment Through Imagery*. Champaign, IL: Human Kinetics.

Grady, Denise. 2002. "Sleep Is One Thing Missing in Busy Teenage Lives." *New York Times*, November 5.

Grieg, Valerie. 1994. *Inside Ballet Technique: Separating Anatomical Fact from Fiction in the Ballet Class*. Hightstown, NJ: Princeton Book Company, Publishers.

Harding, Kelli, MD and Michael Feldman, MD. 2008. "Sleep Disorders and Sleep Deprivation: An Unmet Public Health Problem." *Journal of the American Academy of Child and Adolescent Psychiatry* 47 (4, April): 473–474.

Krasnow, Donna, Gretchen Kerr, and Lynda Mainwaring. 1994. "Psychology of Dealing with the Injured Dancer." *Medical Problems of Performing Artists* 9 (1, March): 7–9.

Maffulli, Nicola, MD, Kai Ming Chan, Rose Macdonald, Robert M. Malina, and Anthony W. Parker. 2001. *Sports Medicine for Specific Ages and Abilities*. London: Harcourt Publishers Limited.

National Highway Traffic Safety Administration (NHTSA). *National Survey of Distracted and Drowsy Driving Attitudes and Behaviors: 2002*. 2002. Vol. 1, Chapter 4. http://www.nhtsa.gov/people/injury/drowsy_driving1/survey-distractive03/drowsy.htm.

Nicholas, J. A. 1975. "Risk Factors, Sports Medicine and the Orthopedic System: An Overview." *Journal of Sports Medicine* 3 (5): 243–259.

Silananda, Sayadaw U. 1995. *The Benefits of Walking Meditation*. Kandy, Sri Lanka: Buddhist Publication Society. http://www.dharmaweb.org/index.php/the-benefits-of-walking-meditation.

Sleep Disorders Help Center. WebMD. http://www.webmd.com/sleep-disorders/default.htm.

United States Department of Labor, Bureau of Labor Statistics. March 1997, 2005 statistics. http://www.bls.gov.

Warren, Michelle, MD. 1999. "Health Issues for Women Athletes: Exercise-Induced Amenorrhea." *The Journal of Clinical Endocrinology and Metabolism* 84 (6): 1892–1896.

2 The Cervical Spine

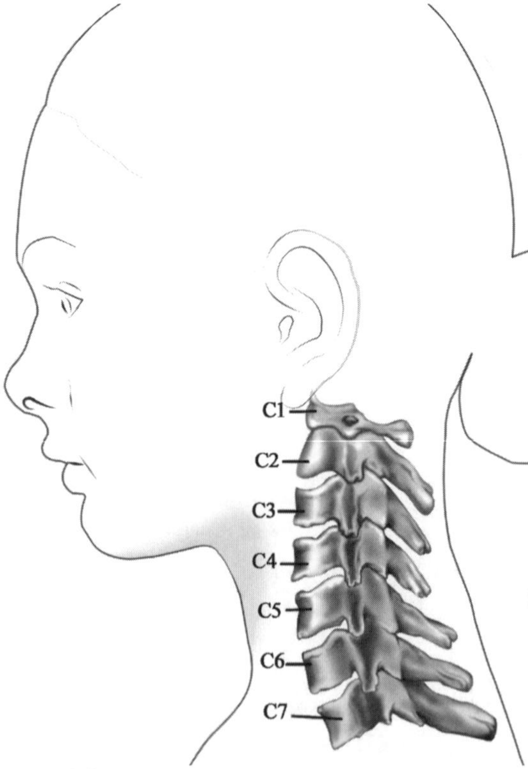

T**HE CERVICAL SPINE IS COMPRISED OF YOUR NECK BONES AND SUPPORTS YOUR SKULL.**

In fact, your skull can be thought of as sitting on the vertebral bones of your neck. There are seven of these vertebral bones in your neck and they are called the cervical vertebral bones. They are numbered as C1 (top neck cervical bone) to C7 (bottom neck cervical bone) (Fig. 2-1).

C1
C2
C3
C4
C5
C6
C7

FIG 2-1

For your head to be able to rotate for spotting, it makes sense that the first two bones of your neck, C1 and C2, would need to be adapted differently from the cervical bones C3 to C7 (Fig. 2-2).

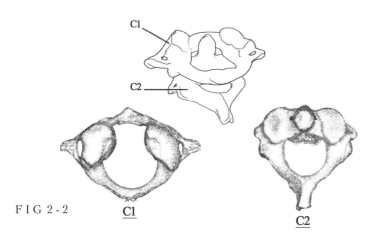

FIG 2-2   C1   C2

THE ATLAS STRENGTH OF THE FIRST NECK BONE (C1)—LOOKING UP

Atlas held up the world on his shoulders in ancient Greek mythology. Similarly, C1, the first bone in your neck, is called the *atlas* bone because it holds up the weight of your skull. And your head is heavy! The average head weighs about eight to twelve pounds. So basically, you are balancing a bowling ball in space on the atlas bone. No wonder dancers get a lot of neck pain if they do extended periods of bending from the waist with cambré! When you look straight up at the ceiling or down to the floor, most of that motion comes from the skull and C1 first vertebral body interface (Fig. 2-3).

FIG 2-3

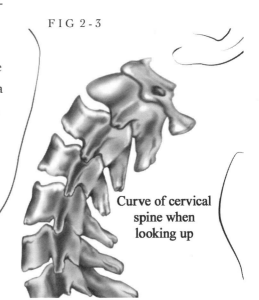

Curve of cervical spine when looking up

Your ability to look up at the ceiling is limited because the bumps at the back of your skull, called the *occipital condyles*, hit the ring of your atlas C1 vertebra and that is as far back as your head will be able to go. No matter how hard you try to force your head back, you will have a fixed point that you cannot move beyond.

How can anyone ever look straight up, then? Dancers vary in their ability to look straight up, yet they all need to give the illusion that they can. As a result, dancers start using compensatory movements. For example, a dancer might make up for lack of movement at the skull and cervical vertebral interface by stretching back their whole neck. The dancer might compensate by flattening the thorax or arching the low back, which, of course, can cause all kinds of strains and neck and back pain. Clinicians who treat dancers are aware of the compensatory movements that many dancers use. Because of this, clinicians familiar with treating dancers will be able to use a more regional approach to treatment that can have better success in keeping them dancing pain free.

THE AXIS (C2)—TAKING A LOOK AROUND

The first cervical bone C1 was called the atlas because it has to be strong to lift your heavy head. C2, the second cervical bone, is called the *axis* bone because your head rotates around the axis of C2. When you whip your head around to spot, a lot of that mobility comes from the C1–C2 interface or *articulation* (Swartz, Floyd, and Cendoma 2005, page 2 of pages 1-11. http://pubmedcental.nih.gov/articlerender.fcgi?artid=1250253). C2 has a spike of bone called the *odontoid peg* that sticks into the atlas or C1 and allows your head to rotate (Fig. 2-4).

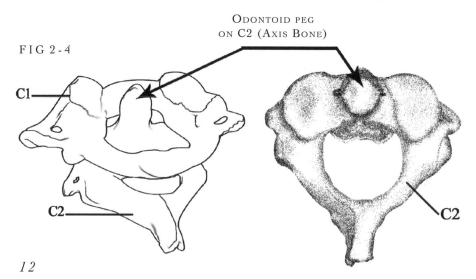

ODONTOID PEG
ON C2 (AXIS BONE)

FIG 2-4

C1

C2

C2

YOUR SPINE AND THE SLINKY TOY

The lower bones of your neck from C3–C7 are curved like a bow. This is the first of a series of spine curves. If you look at yourself in the mirror from the side your low back curves toward your stomach, your mid back curves the opposite way, and your neck is bowed into a curve like your lower spine. You will see these spinal curves even in dancers who hold themselves fairly erect.

These curves allow you to withstand greater loads on your spine without the bones of your back breaking or collapsing. The curves allow your back to store energy like a spring stores energy—as a slinky toy does (Nordin and Weiner 2001, 267). The discs in between the vertebral bones of your neck store some of this energy, too. If your neck is so straight that there is no curve, you will feel the shocks of your landings to a degree that would eventually damage your spine and discs.

The curves of your spine change as you age and your muscles and bones get stronger. But you never completely lose the curves in your spine, because if you did, your risk of injury would increase as your flexibility of movement decreased (Fig. 2-5).

Doctors use the terms *lordosis* and *kyphosis* to describe these curves. Think of spine curves as bowls. If you could pour milk in the bowl from the front, you have a kyphosis. If you would need to pour milk in the bowl from the back you have a lordosis. Your neck has a normal lordosis. Your mid-back or thoracic spine has a normal kyphosis. Your low back has a normal lordosis.

Sometimes dancers will have neck pain and a doctor will check an x-ray to see if the normal curves are present in the neck.

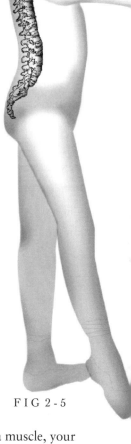

FIG 2-5

If you suddenly lose the curve in your neck after you have pulled a muscle, your x-ray shows a pretty straight spine. Muscles often have to be pulling pretty hard to get your spine curves straight! And that straight neck spine with a flattened curve in the presence of neck pain tells the doctor that you have neck muscle spasms. So even though the doctor cannot see muscles on an x-ray, the x-ray still helps the doctor know what is going on with your muscles.

13

Muscles and nerves

The two large straps that come from the back of your jaw line to the breastbone in front are called the *sternocleidomastoids*. When you turn your head left, the right sternocleidomastoids bulge out and vice versa. When you nod your head down, both sternocleidomastoids fire together to help bring your chin to your chest.

There is another muscle called the *longus colli* which is a long muscle of your neck that sits right in front of upper thoracic and lower cervical vertebral bones and then attaches higher up in the neck and on the C1 atlas. It is the muscle that is most responsible for nodding your head down. This is also a muscle that is frequently injured if your head snaps up and down suddenly from a car crash or a whiplash type injury.

When you look up at the sky, the splenius capitis muscle pulls you back and also rotates your head. The enormous trapezius muscle also works to extend your head by having the upper muscle fibers pull your head backwards. There is a series of dorsal muscles from your back that also extend your head back to look up at your partner in an overhead lift. If your shoulders are stabilized, the *levator scapulae* will extend the neck back (Magee 2002, 138).

The scalene muscles perform a great deal of the work of bending your head to the side. Shoulder pain that seems to follow the inner border of your shoulder blade can be caused by this muscle being overactive and tight (Fig. 2-6).

FIG 2-6

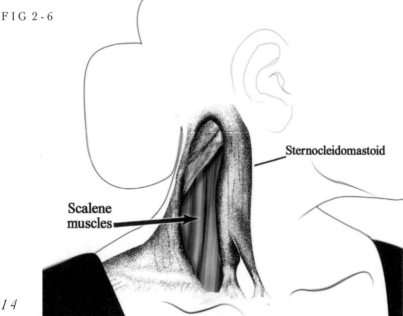

Sternocleidomastoid

Scalene muscles

NECK PAIN
The front of my neck hurts

The front of your neck has your windpipe or *trachea*, your voice box or *larynx*, and the carotid arteries and other major blood vessels. People who have an upper respiratory infection will often notice the lumps and bumps of swollen lymph nodes in the front of their neck. Your esophagus can refer pain to the front of your neck. Your heart can even refer pain to the front of your neck!

Dancers with pain in the front of their necks or persistent swelling need to be checked by a medical doctor to make sure there is not a serious medical condition causing a problem. Many different problems ranging from swallowing issues to a muscle strain can cause front-of-neck pain. I would recommend a medical doctor evaluate this problem of pain before you assume that it is from a strain of your sternocleidomastoid or another muscle. Too many other types of conditions can refer pain to the front of your neck for you to assume on your own that this is a benign and self-limiting type of problem. You should get it checked (Fig. 2-7).

FIG 2-7

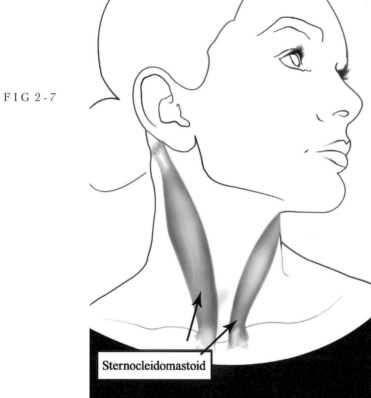

Sternocleidomastoid

Pain on the side of your neck

Pulling a muscle or sudden movements can cause pain on the side of the neck for dancers. I remember walking down the street one day in Philadelphia. I saw one of our dancers from Pennsylvania Ballet walking down the sidewalk holding an ice bag to the side of his neck! This dancer had pulled a muscle in dance class and he had a strain of one muscle on the side of his neck. Because it had just happened, he was correctly trying to rest from class and use ice and compression to try to help his condition. Often rest, moist heat that you can start a day or two after the original muscle pull, and stretching will be all that is necessary to get the symptoms to resolve.

If you are forcing your shoulders down to get that long neck line for dance, you may get pain on the side of your neck and your port de bras may be stiff. Technical correction from your teacher may allow these issues to resolve.

If you feel pain on the side of your neck associated with popping inside your ear or cracking noises of your jaw, you may be experiencing symptoms from the jaw joint called the *temporomandibular joint (TMJ)* (Fig. 2-8).

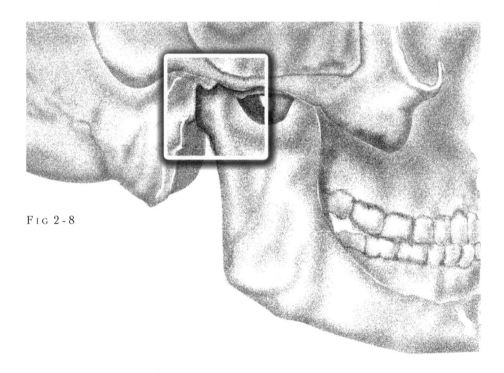

FIG 2-8

Temporomandibular joint pain can make it hurt to open your mouth and can cause a lot of neck discomfort. Often temporomandibular joint pain can be helped a great deal by a few simple changes. If you have TMJ issues, stop eating bagels! Avoid any bread that is toasted and really chewy. Avoid pizza. The high-stress lifestyle of dance can cause tension that contributes to the pain of TMJ. Try to unwind with some relaxation tapes, meditation, music, etc.

Finally, your dentist is a terrific person to help with TMJ. Some dancers grind their teeth at night contributing to TMJ pain and neck pain and headache. A really well-made bite plate can allow the muscles causing the TMJ pain to relax and help solve the pain problem. Bite splints sold over the counter are a less expensive start to getting the problems fixed. A dentist can fabricate a custom bite splint molded to your specific bite pattern that can very helpful for relieving the symptoms of TMJ pain. Warm compresses applied to the cheek back toward the jaw right before you go to sleep also helps to alleviate TMJ pain.

Pain in the back of your neck

Muscles and ligaments in the back of your neck can cause neck pain. In addition, dancers can bang together the joints of the cervical vertebrae—and this can cause neck pain and headache. Most of the time this type of problem is very positional. The dancer feels good until he or she has to turn the head or look up and then— whammo! The dancer experiences pain and aching in the back of the neck that even goes up into the head with a headache.

The discs between the bones of your spine can tear or become injured, causing significant pain and or a very stiff neck. There may be burning tingling or numb pain that goes down the back of the shoulder or even into the arm (Tsang 2001, 1183). Your arm might feel like it is on fire or it might feel weak. This is because the disc is pinching some of the nerves that make up the brachial plexus (which is discussed later in this chapter).

The treatments for disc and brachial plexus problems are different because there is a different site of compression of the nerve in each case. Because of this, dancers with either neck pain and headache or neck pain and tingling should see their medical doctor prior to beginning treatment. Dancers with a disc irritation can benefit from physical therapy, neck isometric exercises, traction which pulls on the discs, acupuncture, and technical training to soften the landings from jumps (Fig. 2-9).

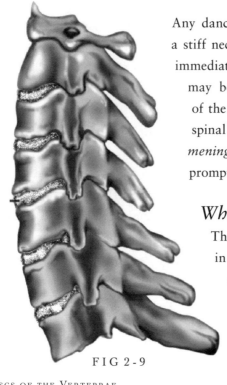

FIG 2-9

DISCS OF THE VERTEBRAE

Any dancer with a stiff neck and a fever or a stiff neck and a headache needs to be seen immediately by a medical doctor because there may be actual infection or inflammation of the tissues that surround the brain and spinal cord. This condition is known as *meningitis*, is extremely serious, and needs prompt medical care.

Whiplash and stiff neck

The classic "whiplash" injury occurs in a motor vehicle crash when another car hits the back end of your car and your head whips forward and back, straining the muscles and injuring the small joints of your neck. Another classic way to get whiplash is in contact sports. The football player is tackled from the back; his head whips forward and back, and he has a whiplash.

Whiplash affects the soft tissues of the neck such as the muscles, ligaments, discs, and nerves. The small joints in the back of your neck where the neck bones link together may get irritated from sudden neck movements. These are facet joints or Z-joints (Z is short for *zygapophyseal*). Your neck may stay stiff for a few days after a whiplash.

Dancers can get whiplash, too! Any sudden movement that stretches the muscles and ligaments of the neck can cause a whiplash-type neck injury. Dancers can suddenly try to force their neck into extension or they may be thrust into the air in a lift but get off balance and whip their neck—either of these actions can result in whiplash. When you whip your head around to spot or suddenly move your neck and you get pain the back of your neck or the big strap muscles that run from your jaw to your collarbone—the sternocleidomastoids—you have a type of whiplash (Kasch, et al. 2001).

Stingers and burners and the brachial plexus

Guess what a stinger or a burner feels like? You're correct! The nerves that go out to our shoulders, arms, and hands get to those areas by first exiting the spinal cord and then passing through tiny holes in the spine called *foramina* (Fig. 2-10).

FIG 2-10

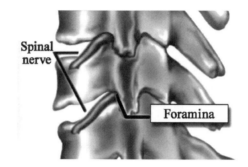

These nerves combine into a network called the *brachial plexus*. The brachial plexus is a bundle of nerves that gives sensation and motor power to your arms. Any movement that stretches your shoulder too far down or turns your chin too far to the side can stretch the nerves. Irritated, stretched nerves feel tingly and burning and hence the term *burner* to describe what is essentially a nerve stretch injury. Dancers who keep their elbows too far back can have this problem also, as this also stretches the brachial plexus as it exits the neck area and goes under the collarbone (Fig. 2-11).

FIG 2-11

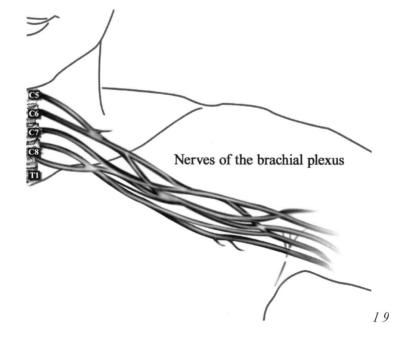

Nerves of the brachial plexus

Dancers who have numb, tingling, weak arms need to be evaluated by a medical doctor. If they have a true stinger or burner caused by the technical problem of leading with the elbow rather than using the correct placement of the elbow and hand, they will often benefit from technical correction. Stretches of the pectoral muscles of the chest wall will be very helpful. Scapular stabilization exercises will help improve the general carriage of the upper torso and also help with brachial plexus stretch injury recovery.

Chronic neck pain and dance

Some dancers have chronic, ongoing neck tightness. Sometimes this chronic neck tightness is because the dancer is forcing the turn-out by swaying the low back and dropping the pelvis in an attempt to make the turn-out look more impressive. It is strange to think that you might have neck pain because of what is happening with your turn-out. However, it all makes sense. If you sway your low back to increase turn-out, you might *compensate* higher in your back. Your thoracic curve would possibly increase and you might change the placement of your head, too, to keep everything in a line (Howse 2000, 178–190).

If you did not do these compensations, your center of gravity would fall in the wrong place and you would be off balance. These compensations momentarily work for the dancer but cause neck and shoulder problems over time. By doing these compensations, you cause carrying tension in your neck and shoulders. This is the reason that problems with forcing the turn-out can cause some dancers to have chronic neck tightness.

Dancers can also have chronic posterior neck tightness because of poor stabilization and endurance in the lower back and trunk muscles. The abdomen is weak; the low back fatigues. The posture starts to slip a little. This dancer with poor core strength will then tense the shoulders and neck in an attempt to hold everything together and in place. This holding tension in the neck and shoulders strains the muscles and fatigues them, causing pain (Howse 2000, 180–181).

Eric Franklin, an expert on movement and imagery, talks about how we need to change our minds to change our bodies. Dancers need to work on positive imagery associations to allow the body to "problem solve." This approach contains a lot of wisdom. If you have danced a piece fifty times and it is going nowhere, the body gets tense and tight. Eric Franklin instead talks about how, if the training is not working, dancers need to be able to create a different choice to allow the movement to occur.

In his book *Dynamic Alignment through Imagery*, Franklin offers a terrific image for helping your spinal alignment. He talks about your spine as a series of spotlights, shining forward as you stand. If the lights are shining all over the place, adjust them so they all shine in one direction. Make them shine equally brightly (Franklin 1996, 192). This simple image will powerfully help your standing posture to be relaxed yet in a true neutral position and not shifted off on one leg because of habit or fatigue. Many dancers with problems getting their hips to be level or their pelvis in the correct position (level, not tucked under, not tipped forward) will be helped with this simple visualization exercise if they simply practice it daily.

> *Remember, "no pain no gain" is not the intelligent way to train in dance. Allowing movements to happen with correct technique and expressivity will be more productive aesthetically and athletically for both your art and your body. Attention to proper technique, working with a physical therapist skilled in treating dancers, and a focus on relaxation of the neck and chest muscles will be helpful. Strengthening the core help, too.*
>
> *Remember that pain is a signal that there might be a problem. Instead of ignoring pain, try to listen to what your body is telling you!*

Dancers with chronic neck pain can often get symptomatic relief from acetaminophen or ibuprofen. A warm neck wrap can really help. Dancers who live in cold climates will want to wear a scarf so their neck muscles do not have to tense up unnecessarily in the cold. Dancers who carry a dance bag that weighs down one shoulder need to rethink this! If you continually stress one shoulder with a heavy dance bag, you may develop asymmetric neck tightness that will eventually give you neck pain. Finally, talk with your doctor and physical therapist about which neck pillow will help the most with your positioning at night so that your neck muscles can relax and recover before the next set of classes.

THE PORTS DE BRAS:

THE CLASSIC ARM POSITIONS OF BALLET

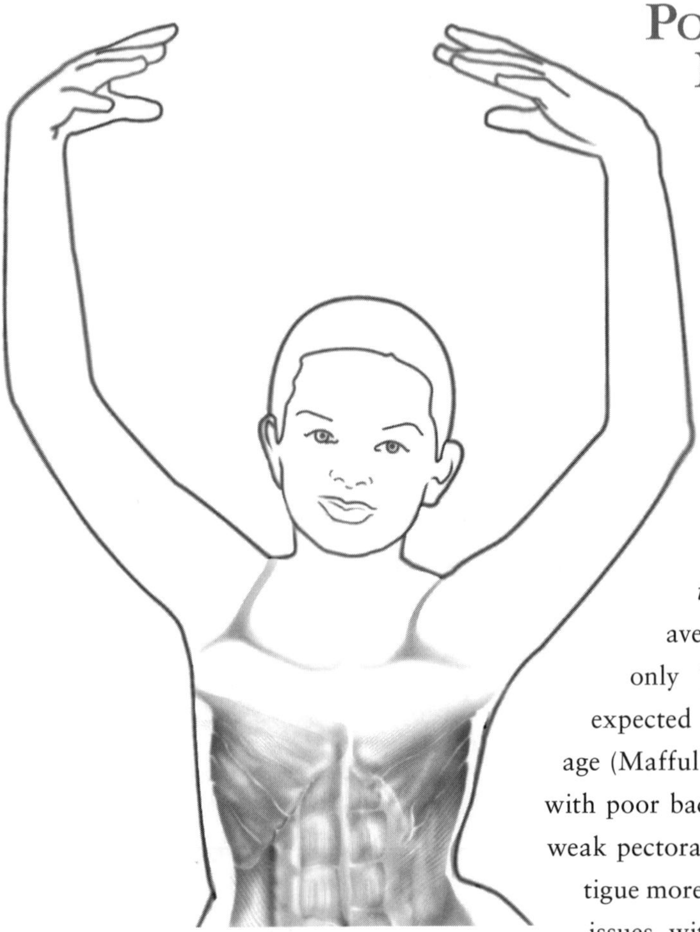

The classic beautiful lines of the port de bras should start from the trunk muscles (Fig. 2-12).

Dancers look strong but the authors of *Sports Medicine for Specific Ages and Abilities* comment that the average ballet dancer has only 77% of the strength expected in people of a similar age (Maffulli et al. 2001). Dancers with poor back muscle strength and weak pectoral chest muscles will fatigue more quickly and have more issues with maintaining proper technique. Strengthening the back muscles and shoulder stabilizers is therefore very important to the development of what would appear to the audience as flowing and graceful movement of the arms. Dancers with neck tightness need to learn to let go so as not to inhibit the movement of the arms. Dancers with tightness because of technical issues with turn-out, weak back, or leading the port de bras with their elbows can get help from a dance medicine specialist and their teacher.

FIG 2-12

MUSCLES OF THE TRUNK

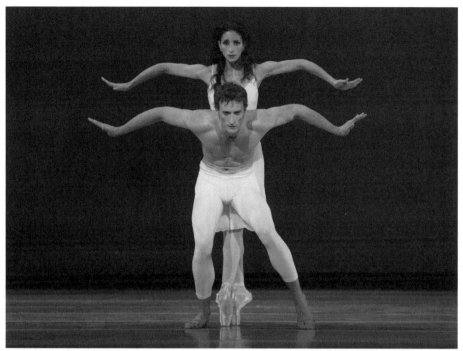

PENNSYLVANIA BALLET PRINCIPAL DANCER RIOLAMA LORENZO AND COMPANY MEMBER MAXIMILIEN BAUD IN PETER MARTINS'S *BARBER VIOLIN CONCERTO*. PHOTOGRAPH BY ALEXANDER IZILIAEV.

Five Critical Issues to Know About Your Neck

1. A good port de bras begins with strong back muscles.

2. Chronic neck tension can lead to chronic neck pain. Imagery can help.

3. Tingling, numbness, and weakness in your arm may be a burner from the brachial plexus or a disc irritating a nerve and need to be checked by a medical doctor.

4. Your head is heavy; your neck needs to be strong. Most of us probably are not sufficiently exercising these muscles so they do not become overworked and fatigued.

5. Any dancer with a stiff neck and a fever or a stiff neck and a headache needs to be seen immediately by a medical doctor because there may be actual infection or inflammation of the tissues that surround the brain and spinal cord. This condition is known as *meningitis*, is extremely serious, and needs prompt medical care.

Five Great Neck Exercises

1. Neck isometrics: hold the front of your head so it cannot move; press forward and hold for a count of twenty. Repeat for the back. Repeat for the sides. Do this in the morning and at night.

2. Stretch your right ear toward your right shoulder until you feel a gentle stretch. Stop, rest there,

3. and count to ten. See if you can stretch slightly further and count to ten again. Repeat on the other side.

4. With your head in neutral, rotate your chin toward your shoulder; count to twenty. Repeat on the other side.

5. Inhale and bring your shoulders up toward your ear; exhale and bring your shoulders down—gently and without feeling pushing or strain in the trapezius. Inhale and bring your hands in front of you. Exhale and bring your arms out to the sides. Focus on not allowing your shoulder blades to wing out in the back; keep them pressed against your back. Repeat ten times.

6. Get into a push-up position or modified push-up position on your knees. Lift one hand off and place it on top of the one hand still down on the mat. Repeat with the other hand. Try to work up to sets of five with good shoulder positioning.

References

Franklin, Eric. *Dynamic Alignment Through Imagery.* Champaign, IL: Human Kinetics, 1996.

Howse, Justin. *Dance Technique and Injury Prevention,* 3rd edition. New York, NY: Routledge, 2000.

Kasai, Tokio M.D., Takaaki Ikata, M.D., Shinsuke Katoh, M.D., Ryoji Miyake, M.D. and Masahiko Tsubo, M.D. "Growth of the Cervical Spine with Special Reference to Its Lordosis and Mobility." *Spine* 21, no. 18 (September 1996): 2067–2073.

Kasch, Helge M.D., Ph.D, Kristian Stengaard-Pedersen, M.D, DMSc, Lars Arendt-Nielsen, DMSc and Troels Staehelin Jensen, M.D., DMSc. "Headache, Neck Pain, and Neck Mobility After Acute Whiplash Injury: A Prospective Study." *Spine* 26, no. 11 (June 2001): 1246–1251.

Kuhlman, G. S. and D. B. McKeag. "The 'Burner': A Common Nerve Injury in Contact Sports." *American Family Physician* 60, no. 7 (Nov 1999): 2035–40, 2042.

Magee, David J. *Orthopedic Physical Assessment,* 4th edition. Philadelphia, PA: 2002.

Mafulli, Nicola, M.D., Kai Ming Chan, Rose Macdonald, Robert M. Malina and Anthony W. Parker. *Sports Medicine for Specific Ages and Abilities.* London, UK: Harcourt, 2001.

National Institute of Health. National Institute of Neurologic Disorders and Stroke Whiplash Information Page, http://www.ninds.nih.gov/disorders/whiplash/whiplash.htm.

Nordin, Margareta and Shira Schecter Weiner (adapted from Margareta Lindh). "*Biomechanics of the Lumbar Spine.*" In *Basic Biomechanics of the Musculoskeletal System,* 3rd edition, edited by Margareta Nordin and Victor H. Frankel. Philadelphia, PA: Lippincott, Williams and Wilkins, 2001.

Prisk, Victor R. M.D., and William G. Hamilton, M.D. "Stress Fractures of the Rib in Weight-Trained Dancers." *American Journal of Sports Medicine* 36, no. 12 (December 2008): 2444-2447.

Roach, Mary. Stiff: The Curious Lives of Human Cadavers. New York, NY: Norton Publishers, 2003.

Swartz, Erik E., R. T. Floyd and Mike Cendoma. "Cervical Spine Functional Anatomy and the Biomechanics of Injury Due to Compressive Loading." *Journal of Athletic Training* 40, no. 3 (2005): 155–161.

Tsang, Ian. "Rheumatology: 12. Pain in the neck." *Canadian Medical Association Journal* 164, no. 8 (April 2001): 1182–1187.

3 Thoracic Spine

THORACIC SPINE ANATOMY

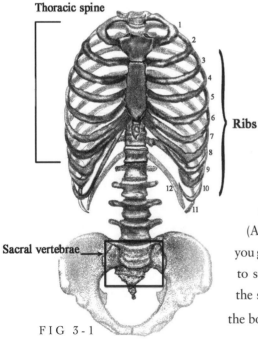

Thoracic spine

Ribs

1
2
3
4
5
6
7
8
9
10
11
12

Sacral vertebrae

FIG 3-1

THE THORACIC SPINE IS DIFFERENT FROM THE CERVICAL SPINE OR THE LUMBAR SPINE. ONLY YOUR MID-BACK THORACIC AREA HAS RIBS THAT COME OUT FROM THE SPINE.

Your cervical neck bones and your lumbar, low back bones are not attached to any type of rib that comes out horizontally (Adamo et al. 2006). You need to wait until you get all the way down to your sacral vertebrae to see any kind of structure coming out from the spine and the structure that is attached are the bones of your pelvis (Fig. 3-1).

26

Your ribs attach to your thoracic spine with joints called costotransverse joints. Costo means rib and transverse means to go across (Fig. 3-2).

The twelve thoracic vertebrae in the zone in between your neck and your low back have ribs, but not all ribs are the same! The ribs near your collarbone are fairly horizontal. You can check this by pressing on the bone underneath your collarbone. It is basically flat. The lower ribs are tilted. You can check this also by feeling along a lower rib (Fig. 3-3).

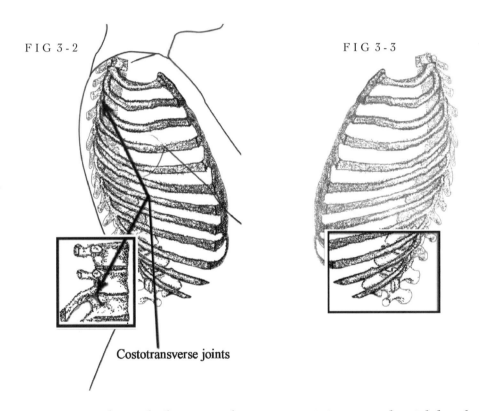

FIG 3-2

FIG 3-3

Costotransverse joints

Open-pack and close-pack joint positions and mid-back mobility

Joints vary in mobility depending upon their position. If you straighten your knee and then try to push your thigh and your lower leg in opposite directions from side to side, they simply do not go. Your leg and thigh stay in a straight line. If you bend your knee and then try the same thing, pushing your thigh and your lower leg in opposite directions, you will feel a little bit of give and your leg will be able to be swing side to side in opposite directions a small amount compared to your thigh. This is because the knee joint has different looseness and mobility in different positions. This concept of a joint having better freedom to move in different positions is called the *open-pack* position of the joint versus the *close-pack* position of the joint. In the close-pack position, the joint cannot move as freely.

The concept of open-pack and close-pack joint positions also applies to the ribs. Because your ribs attach to your thoracic spine with joints, the mobility of your thoracic spine will vary. The rib costotransverse joints have open-pack and close-pack positions, as follows: when you extend your arm back in cambré, your ribs and thoracic spine joints get into a close-pack position and you will have less thoracic rotation] If your choreography calls for a lot of cambré and you are not lifting your ribcage correctly or if your neck is too stiff, you will get rib or mid-back pain.

The rib cage

Your ribs allow your thoracic spine to withstand more force. The heads of some of the thoracic ribs connect in front to your breastbone or sternum in a ring. The thoracic spine and ribs form a ring that connects to your breastbone that is somewhat stiff. This ring of your ribs and spine protects the contents of your thorax, which include your heart and lungs. Because the heart and lungs are so important, it makes a lot of sense that those organs would need to be well protected.

The front of the box of your thorax is formed by the sternum or breastbone; the sides, by the ribs; and the back, by your thoracic vertebrae (Fig. 3-4).

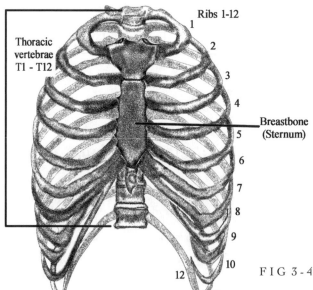

Ribs 1-12

Thoracic vertebrae T1 - T12

1
2
3
4
5
6
7
8
9
10
11
12

Breastbone (Sternum)

FIG 3-4

When you breathe, your ribs move. When you take a deep breath and inhale, your lungs fill and the ribs move up and out to accommodate the increased volume of your lungs. When you exhale, your lungs decrease in volume and your ribs then move down. The external intercostal muscles elevate the ribs for the deep breath of inspiration. The internal intercostals pull the ribs down for the big "whoosh" sound of forced expiration. So when you breathe, there is a lot going on in your thorax, even just between your ribs, in terms of muscular activity.

When you have a bad upper respiratory infection, and you are coughing a lot, your chest wall gets sore and you can actually fracture a rib. This happens because the muscles in between the ribs get a real workout when you have a cough! And all of the pulling of these muscles can cause a fatigue fracture of your rib. The external intercostal muscles elevate the ribs for the deep breath of inspiration. The internal intercostals pull the ribs down for the big "whoosh" sound of forced expiration.

PROBLEMS OF THE THORAX
My teacher says my mid-back is too stiff!

Do you know why something is called a cage? Because it limits movement!

In the front you are working against a rib cage that limits your movement (Gevirtz 2009), and in the back there are long processes that come off the thoracic spine that also limit movement. Every dancer is different, but if you cannot extend back smoothly, without deviating off to the side, there is a problem. You should be able to go into a 25–45 degree backbend without breaking a sweat. If you cannot do this, you will substitute with cervical neck movements or get the range from the low back or your hips—and you will look stiff and unbalanced. As a result, you need to work on this with your dance teacher and physical therapist.

Sometimes the stiffness happens because a rib is stuck in an elevated position (cannot move when you exhale); sometimes stiffness happens because a rib is stuck in a depressed position (cannot move when you inhale); sometimes the stiffness is in the spine itself. A qualified dance medicine doctor can help you figure it out so you regain some mobility.

Scheuermann's Disease

Some teenagers who develop mid-back pain and mid-back stiffness may actually have a condition called *Scheuermann's disease* or *Sherman's disease*. Below is an MRI image of Scheuermann's disease, side view.

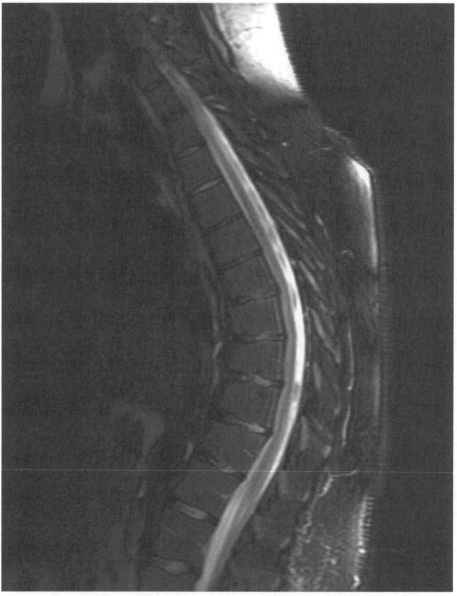

MRI IMAGE COURTESY THOMAS JEFFERSON UNIVERSITY HOSPITAL, PHILADELPHIA, PA.

You can see that the series of bones in the spine do not have the nice straight look of a dancer's back. The bones are pressed together and there is a forward curve. The stiffness in the thoracic spine is caused by a series of compression injuries to the bones that causes the stiffness and the forward bend of the spine (Kim and Green 2008). The dancer with Scheuermann's disease has a rounded back and simply cannot flatten out or reverse the curve on cambré or back extension. Dancers who cannot get into a full back bend may actually have this spine problem. Dancers with Scheuermann's kyphosis will have problems with thoracic extension, mid-back pain, and hamstring tightness. This condition seems to become evident in the teenage years. Perhaps up to 8% of the population may be affected. It seems to run in some families and to more commonly affect boys (Nowak 2009). The dancer appears to have a forward stoop to the shoulders and the spine is curved forward. The dancer may compensate with low back hyperextension that then causes complaints of low back pain.

Dancers with Scheuermann's kyphosis need to be monitored to see if the thoracic forward-directed curve is getting worse. Some dancers may need braces and a change in activity. Remember, if you have a thoracic kyphosis you may develop a compensatory lumbar lordosis. It is very important to have a good strengthening program for all of your trunk muscles. The "slinky" spring of your back is not as good at shock absorption, so you need stronger muscles to help absorb the energy of leaps and landings in dance.

THE THORACOLUMBAR JUNCTION

Even a normal thoracic spine is somewhat limited in its movement by the rib cage and the thoracic spine processes. However, the thoracolumbar junction has significant mobility. The ribcage stops above the lowest ribs. The lowest ribs are floating ribs—they are not attached into the thoracosternal box we talked about earlier. If you feel your sides you feel the ends of these floating ribs (Fig. 3-5).

FIG 3-5

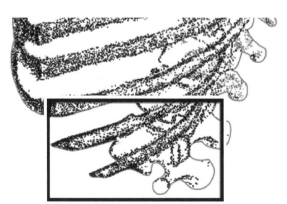

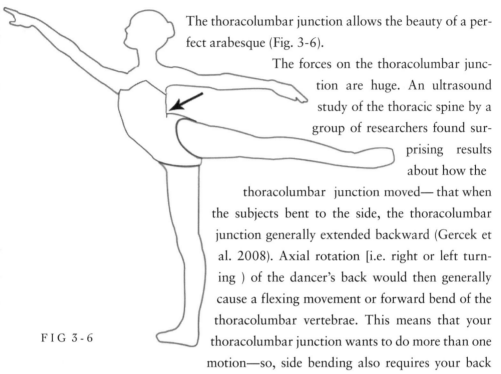

The thoracolumbar junction allows the beauty of a perfect arabesque (Fig. 3-6).

The forces on the thoracolumbar junction are huge. An ultrasound study of the thoracic spine by a group of researchers found surprising results about how the thoracolumbar junction moved— that when the subjects bent to the side, the thoracolumbar junction generally extended backward (Gercek et al. 2008). Axial rotation [i.e. right or left turning) of the dancer's back would then generally cause a flexing movement or forward bend of the thoracolumbar vertebrae. This means that your thoracolumbar junction wants to do more than one motion—so, side bending also requires your back to lengthen or extend. And thoracolumbar rotation requires your back to curve forward or flex. Basically this means that many dance movements of your thoracolumbar junction involve rotation along with bending—and these rotational forces then put extra stress on the thoracolumbar junction.

FIG 3-6

Lifts and thoracolumbar stress

When dancers lift their partners overhead there is tremendous stress at the thoracolumbar region. Dr. K. Peter Gill and his colleagues analyzed the motion of the thoracolumbar spine with different styles of lifting. Eight people lifted a crate weighing approximately 20 pounds (10 kg.) ten times. The person doing the action lifted by squatting (bent knees), stooping (straight knees), or freestyle (whatever the person felt like doing to lift the box). The researchers found that the mid-thoracic spine and thoracolumbar junction were the most affected by the changes in lifting style or box position (Gill et al. 2007).

If you would like a simple illustration of this principle, take a heavy book, hold it three inches in front of your stomach, and then lift it up over your head. Now take that same book, hold it at arm's length away from your stomach, and lift it over your head. Pay attention to what you are feeling in your spine. The forces are hugely different with a lift that is held far away from you.

Partnering is tricky business! The dancer doing the lift has to pay attention to performing the lift by using lumbar, leg, and hip strength, and not just shoulder and arm strength. Think physics. It makes sense that if you decrease the distance between you and your partner and hold him or her close when you lift, you will decrease the forces on your spine.

THE NORMAL THORACIC CURVE

Dancers are also taught to "lengthen the spine." Functionally this means that many dancers try to flatten the normal spine curves. Flattening the curves to lengthen the spine, however, decreases the shock absorbing capacity of the spine. Think about it—making your back one long stiff pipe to jump and land causes huge forces to be transmitted up and down the spine. On the other hand, if there are the normal curves present in the spine, the forces can dissipate, which translates into less potential for injury to the spinal discs, joints, and ligaments. Remember the slinky toy!

Some dancers try to increase their available turnout by overarching their lumbar spine. If you cause your lower back to sway, the turnout at your hips increases. These dancers then compensate for the extreme low back curve with another curve— by overarching the thoracic spine forward. A back that is too stiff causes problems, but a back that is too curved forward and back like an "S" causes stress on the discs as well! If you are a dancer who is arching your low back to increase your turnout, you need to work with your dance teacher and physical therapist to prevent a whole cascade of problems that occur because of this problem with your technique.

Abnormal thoracic curves—scoliosis and the dancer's spine

Some individuals may develop a thoracic curve to the side. This called a *scoliosis*.

There are different types of scoliosis curves. Curves can be a single curve or a double curve. Most of the time scoliosis is seen as a single curve in the thoracic area. If the curve is convex to the right it is called a *dextroscoliosis* and if the curve is convex to the left it is called a *levoscoliosis*.

Some people believe that more time dancing increases the risk of the development of this scoliosis curve developing. Taller height and lower weight were once thought to be risk factors for developing adolescent idiopathic scoliosis. Most doctors now do not believe this to be the case. Some doctors thought that if a person were very strongly right-handed, or left-handed, this would increase the risk of scoliosis—also likely not true! Genetics do play a role—if your mother has scoliosis your risk of developing scoliosis is higher—but there is no simple formula to predict whether or not you might get scoliosis.

However, we do know that if your menstrual period is delayed or if you simply do not ever get a normal menstrual period, your risk of scoliosis increases. Whether or not exercising a great deal is itself a cause of scoliosis remains unknown (Kenanidis et al. 2008). A study of ballet dancers published in the journal *Medical Problems of Performing Artists* examined fifty four ballet dancers who volunteered to participate. A whopping 40.7% had scoliosis curves on physical examination. The researchers found that dancers who had a history of more stress fractures were at higher risk (Akella et al. 1991). Previous studies also found a quite increased risk of scoliosis in ballet dancers, although it is unclear what factors contribute to this finding.

Scoliosis does not mean that you cannot dance. But if you have scoliosis you need to be very careful about your food and calcium intake. If you have scoliosis, you will need to spend extra time stretching your back muscles and your hamstring muscles. Strengthening of your leg and foot musculature will be helpful, too. Remember, if you have a curve, it may be harder for you to find your center in dance. Strong leg and foot muscles and attention to balance exercises will be very helpful to insure that your positioning stays correct and that you do not compensate by tightening your shoulders and neck. Finally, your doctor

DEXTROSCOLIOSIS

needs to evaluate you to see if there is a medical condition that is causing your curve, such as a spine fracture or any other serious medical condition. Most of the time, though, there is no known reason why some people get scoliosis.

Mild scoliosis (less than 20 degrees of angle of the vertebral bones to each other by a special measurement done by the radiology doctor who reviews your x-ray) is usually not painful, but all patients with scoliosis need to be monitored. Scoliosis curves can get bigger, particularly if you are still growing. This can cause a problem with your general body symmetry, which makes sense because your spine is curved to the side. It can cause hip and back pain if the curves get large. Very large curves can even affect your breathing.

If you have scoliosis, pay close attention to how you carry a book bag or dance bag. Try to switch shoulders back and forth. Correct stretching exercise can also help all dancers with mild scoliosis curves get less back tightness and have better symmetry. Do shoulder stretches and side stretches, such as a daily stretch of bending to the side with your arm overhead pointing away from the apex of your curve. Finally, Marika Molnar, a physical therapist with many years of experience treating dancers at all levels of training, was asked about scoliosis for an article in *Dance Magazine*. Molnar suggested breathing exercises as being helpful for many of the dancers she saw with spinal scoliosis. Breathing exercises will help your chest cage expansion and help relax your back muscles.

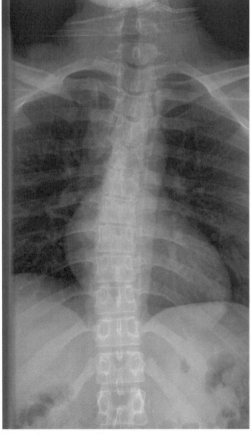

MILD SCOLIOSIS. X-RAY IMAGE COURTESY OF THOMAS JEFFERSON UNIVERSITY HOSPITAL, PHILADELPHIA, PA.

Just remember to get your scoliosis curve checked at least yearly!

THORACIC DISCS

Symptomatic thoracic disc herniation in a general population of non-dancers is really felt to be a pretty uncommon occurrence (Hoffmeister 2005). As a matter of fact, maybe one or two out of a hundred symptomatic disc herniations in a general population are thought to be secondary to a disc herniation in the thoracic spine area. Dancers, of course, are not anything like a general population. The general population does not lift women overhead throughout the workday! Dancers' thoracolumbar and thoracic spine health is at risk because of the forces present in dance.

Most thoracic disc herniations are found below T7, in the lower thoracic region (Gevirtz 2009). Your ribs 8, 9, and 10 connect to your breastbone by cartilage that can bend and move. Ribs 11 and 12 are not attached to any bony structure—not even through cartilage—and these lower ribs are able to move as you bend and twist (Fig. 3-7).

This greater amount of movement in the lower thoracic spine, which can torque and tear the outer part of the disc, probably at least partly explains why the inner part of the lower thoracic discs are more at risk of herniation. Once the disc material bulges out of place, it can impinge on nerves and cause pain and problems.

FIG. 3-7

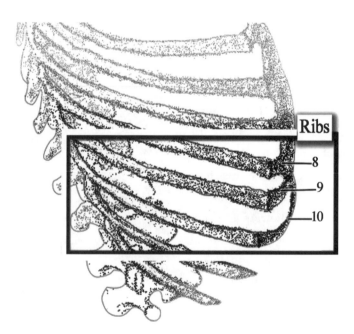

Ribs
8
9
10

Dancers who feel a pop in their back after a lift and then have pain need to be checked by a medical doctor for a disc problem. Dancers who experience numbness, tingling, electric sensations, weakness, or bladder urgency after performing a lift need to get checked by a medical doctor immediately for a thoracic disc injury (Baranto et al. 2009).

First rib injuries in dancers

The first rib gets a workout in dance! Turning your head to spot for a pirouette pulls on the first rib (Fig. 3-8).

The neck muscles called the *scalenes* pull up on the first rib (see Fig. 2-6) and the shoulder muscle called the *serratus* anterior pulls down on the first rib. Dancers who are experiencing neck, collarbone, or shoulder pain who are doing a great deal of pirouette work or lifts may actually have a stress fracture of the first rib. Dancers who have neck or shoulder pain with dance need to be evaluated by a physician experienced in dance medicine. Stress fractures that are not treated by adequate rest take longer to heal and are more painful. Also, there may be a problem with your general bone health. Dancers with weak bones or

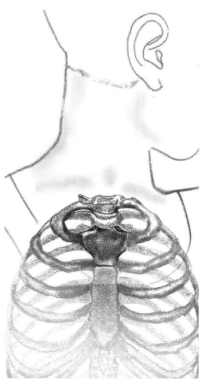

FIG. 3-8

low calcium are a setup for stress fractures. A doctor can help treat the underlying bone health issue and this treatment will then decrease the chances that you get future additional stress fractures because of weak bones.

The lower ribs also can get injured in dance

To lift a dancer overhead takes a lot of strength and stability. Positioning is not always perfect and costuming can make the task even more difficult. Those bulky bodices and slippery tulles can make it harder to do the lift. The lifting partner may have to use a lot of force to make sure his or her partner is not dropped on stage! This lifting force can cause stress on the lower ribs. One study showed tiny micro-fractures on both sides of the lower ribcage in a dancer who was being checked for problems with leg pain (Bar-Sever, Connolly, and Treves 1997). If you are someone who gets a lot of stress fractures and you have rib pain or trunk pain, you could have stress fractures of these lower ribs. Any kind of torso pain, chest wall discomfort, tightness of breathing, or pain that is worse with a deep breath—could be a rib fracture, another serious medical condition like asthma, or a lung problem that needs treatment. So get yourself checked by a doctor. And remember to thank your partner for holding on tight because, most of the time, rib stress fractures are still a lot better than being dropped on the studio floor!

Slipped lower ribs in dancers

You do continuous fouetté turns. And you do them again. And then again to really get them right. And then your ribs hurt. The floating ribs (ribs 11 and 12) may actually have moved out of place and slipped. The movement and sliding of the ribs can aggravate the rib nerves and muscles. This situation is called a *slipped rib*.

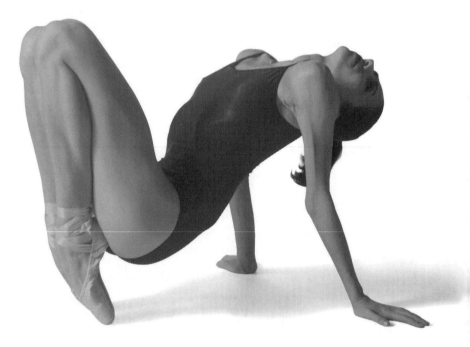

ARANTXA OCHOA, PENNSYLVANIA BALLET PRINCIPAL DANCER. PHOTOGRAPH BY STEVE BELKOWITZ.

Ribs out of place in dancers

Some dancers are told by their health professionals that a rib has jumped out of place (Udermann et al. 2005). The dancer has mid-back pain or pain in the front. Ribs 8, 9, or 10 are usually involved—roughly middorsal back. Movement is painful and the dancer's back is very sore. A forceful movement by the dancer has likely torn the ligaments that hold the rib in place near the spine. This is called a *costovertebral subluxation* (Sik, Batt, and Heslop 2009). As we noted earlier, some ribs can get stuck and not move in a correctly coordinated way with the ribs around them when the dancer inhales with a deep breath in or exhales and breathes out.

Manipulation treatment with chiropractic or physical therapy will help get the rib seated correctly again. Over time, and with rest and anti-inflammatory medication, the pain will settle down and the ligaments will heal. Dancers with tight thoracic muscles can help themselves with breathing and relaxation exercises that will improve thoracic mobility and help stretch the muscles in between the ribs.

Five Important Things to Know about Your Thoracic Spine and Ribs

1. Your thoracic spine has a normal forward curve or kyphosis and a lumbar backward curve or lordosis. If the thoracic spine is too straight or too arched forward, you need to be checked for thoracic spine or rib problems.

2. If your spine is curved to the side, the condition is called scoliosis. Many dancers have scoliosis. Having scoliosis does not mean that you cannot dance. But you do need to have your thoracic scoliosis curve monitored by a medical professional.

3. Dancers with low bone mass and delayed menstrual periods have an increased risk of scoliosis.

4. Scoliosis can be helped with exercises to keep muscles in the back relaxed and stretched.

5. Dancers with chest wall pain may have rib injuries that should get checked so they do not get worse.

Five Great Exercises and Stretches for the Thoracic Spine

1. Squeeze your shoulder blades together, count to five, release. Do three sets of ten repetitions about three times a day.

2. Put a broom or stick behind your shoulders. Loop your forearms over the stick and slowly twist back and forth about ten times.

3. Link your hands behind you and stretch back. You should feel a nice long pull. Count to fifteen or twenty and then release.

4. Do a stretch by standing with your feet shoulder-width apart and rotate your torso. Don't force the movement and feel a gentle stretch. Keep your pelvis level while you are standing. Repeat on the other side. Stand with both arms overhead. Grab your left elbow with your right hand and pull to feel the stretch. Repeat on the other side.

References

Adamo, Matthew A., Eric M. Deshaies, John W. German, Darryl J. DiRisio, and John A. Popp. 2006. "Management of Thoracic Spine Injuries, Part 1: Thoracic Spine Anatomy and Stability." *Contemporary Neurosurgery* 28 (20, October): 1–5.

Akella, Priya, Michelle P. Warren, Suhasini Jonnavithula, and J. Brooks-Gunn. 1991 "Scoliosis in Ballet Dancers." *Medical Problems of Performing Artists* 6 (3, September): 84–86.

Auvinen, Juha P., Tuija H. Tammelin, Simo P. Taimela, Paavo J. Zitting, Pertti O. A. Mutanen, and Jaro I. Karppinen. 2008. "Musculoskeletal Pains in Relation to Different Sport and Exercise Activities in Youth." *Medicine and Science in Sport and Exercise* 40 (11, November): 1890–1900.

Baranto, Adad, Mats Börjesson, Barbro Danielsson, Mikael Hellström, and Lief Swärd. 2009. "Acute Chest Pain in a Top Soccer Player Due to Thoracic Disc Herniation." *Spine* 34 (10, May): E359–E362.

Bar-Sever, Zvi, Leonard P. Connolly, and S. Ted Treves. 1997. "Stress Changes in the Ribs Associated with Ballet Dancing." *Clinical Nuclear Medicine* 22 (4, April): 263–264.

Gercek, Erol, Frank Hartmann, Sebastian Kuhn, Jurgen Degreif, Pol Maria Rommens, and Lothat Rudig. 2008. "Dynamic Angular Three-Dimensional Measurement of Multisegmental Thoracolumbar Motion in Vivo." *Spine* 33 (21, October): 2326–2333.

Gevirtz, Clifford. 2009 "Pain Management of the Patient with Thoracic Disc Herniation." *Topics in Pain Management* 24 (6, January): 1–6

Gill, K. Peter, PhD; Simon J. Bennett, PhD; Geert J. P. Savelsbergh, PhD; and Jaap H. van Dieën, PhD. 2007. "Regional Changes in Spine Posture at Lift Onset with Changes in Lift Distance and Lift Style." *Spine* 32 (15, July): 1599–1604.

Hoffmeister, Ellen. 2005. "Thoracic Herniated Discs: Diagnosis is Key." *Bone and Joint* 11 (11, December): 121, 123, 124–125.

Kenanidis, Eustathios, Michael E. Potoupnis, Kyrakios A. Papavasiliou, Fares E. Sayegh, and George A. Kapetanos. 2008. "Adolescent Idiopathic Scoliosis and Exercising: Is There Truly a Liaison?" *Spine* 33 (20, September): 2160–2165.

Kim, Han Jo and Daniel W. Green. 2008. "Adolescent Back Pain." *Current Opinion in Pediatrics* 20 (1, February): 37–45.

Kim, Okumura. 2006. "Health and Fitness: Thrown a Curve: On Conquering Scoliosis." *Dance Magazine* (October). http://www.thefreelibrary.com/Health+and+fitness%3a+thrown+a+curve%3a +on+conquering+scoliosis.-a0152433175.

Kruse, David and Brooke Lemmen. 2009. "Spine Injuries in the Sport of Gymnastics." *Current Sports Medicine Reports* 8 (1, January/February): 20–28.

Nowak, Jozef E. 2009. "Scheuermann Disease." *EMedicine from WebMD.com.* Article updated April 2. http://emedicine.medscape.com/article/311959-overview.

Prisk, Victor R. and William G. Hamilton. 2008. "Stress Fracture of the First Rib in Weight-Trained Dancers." *The American Journal Sports Medicine* 36 (12): 2444–2447.

Schiller, Jonathan R., MD, and Craig P. Eberson, MD. 2008. "Spinal Deformity and Athletics." *Sports Medicine and Arthroscopy Review* 16 (1, March): 26–31.

Sik, Emma C., Mark E. Batt, and Laurence M. Heslop. 2009. "Atypical Chest Pain in Athletes." *Current Sports Medicine Reports* 8 (2, March/April): 0–6.

Udermann, Brian E., Daniel G. Cavanaugh, Mark H. Gibson, Scott T. Doberstein, John M. Mayer, and Steven R Murray. 2005. "Slipping Rib Syndrome in a Collegiate Swimmer: A Case Report." *Journal of Athletic Training* 40 (2, April–June): 120–122.

Warren, Michelle P., MD; J. Brooks Gunn, PhD; Linda H. Hamilton; L. Fiske Warren, MD; and William G. Hamilton, MD. 1986. "Scoliosis and Fractures in Young Ballet Dancers—Relationship to Delayed Menarche and Secondary Amenorrhea." *New England Journal of Medicine* 314: 1348–1353.

Wood, K. B., T. A. Garvey, C. Gundry, and K. B. Heithoff. 1995. "Magnetic Resonance Imaging of the Thoracic Spine: Evaluation of Asymptomatic Individuals." *Journal of Bone and Joint Surgery* 77 (11): 1631–1638.

4 The Lung, The Heart and Dance

Y OU TAKE A DEEP BREATH. A LARGE MUSCLE CALLED THE DIAPHRAGM IN YOUR CHEST CONTRACTS. THE MUSCLES BETWEEN YOUR RIBS CALLED THE INTERCOSTALS CONTRACT. THE PRESSURE IN YOUR CHEST DROPS AND YOUR LUNGS FILL WITH AIR.

BREATHING ALLOWS YOUR BODY TO RID ITSELF OF EXCESS CARBON DIOXIDE AND INSTEAD GET OXYGEN. THE OXYGEN ALLOWS YOUR BRAIN AND MUSCLES TO FUNCTION PROPERLY.

ASTHMA

Asthma is a medical term for a condition in which your breathing can get intermittently more difficult because your airways narrow (Fig. 4-1).

A good way to see what this feels like is to sit down and take a deep breath. Now take a soda straw, and try breathing in and out a few times through the straw.

It is much harder to breathe because the airway is narrower. As you can see, if you have asthma and you are trying to dance, you would need to make certain that your asthma was well controlled!

Asthma is common. Probably about one in ten people in the general population will have asthma. Robert Joffrey, the founder of the Joffrey Ballet, struggled with asthma. He stated that he actually started dancing because his doctors thought it might help his asthma and his asthma certainly did not stop him from pursuing a very successful dance career (Anawalt 1996, 24).

Because asthma reversibly narrows the tubes in your respiratory system, asthma attacks make it hard for people to breathe properly. When people do not breathe properly, they feel fatigued; they feel chest tightness; they cough and they wheeze.

Asthma varies in how severely it affects people. Some people can have very severe attacks. There are 4,000 deaths a year in the United States from asthma. If you have asthma, it is very important to work with your doctor to keep your asthma symptoms under control so they do not interfere with your activities.

Dance and movement can trigger asthma attacks. Some people who usually do not have a breathing problem will get asthma attacks when they exercise. This is another type of asthma—exercise-induced—that happens only after exercise and is distinct from the more common asthma. Exercise-induced asthma means that your airways narrow and constrict when you exercise (see Fig. 4-1). You might have

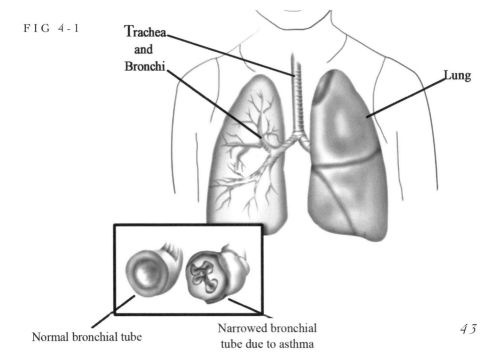

FIG 4-1

Trachea and Bronchi

Lung

Normal bronchial tube

Narrowed bronchial tube due to asthma

exercise-induced asthma if you easily get out of breath with exercise, if you cough after exercise, if you feel winded as if you cannot catch your breath after exercise, if you wheeze after exercise, or your chest feels tight. You need to be checked for exercise-induced bronchospasm and asthma.

Decreasing the impact of asthma

Living in a smoky environment can make asthma symptoms worse. Smog and air pollution are also not good for people with asthma. If a studio frequently has animals in it or is dusty, that can make asthma worse. A dance studio that is freezing cold, bone dry, or swelteringly hot may also make breathing more difficult. Air-conditioned studios are helpful, however, because there may be fewer temperature swings and less exposure to smog and pollen from the outside.

Additionally, many researchers think stress can trigger asthma attacks. Stress reduction techniques and relaxation techniques may help some dancers with control of their asthma symptoms.

The better your general conditioning and the better your health is overall will have an impact on how your asthma affects you.

Tobacco use

Smoking tobacco is a very bad idea for any dancer, but is particularly bad for any dancer with a history of asthma.

Tobacco use continues to be a problem among dancers. Actually, tobacco use is a common problem among all teenagers! Nine percent of high school seniors in the United States are thought to regularly use tobacco (Pumariega and Hashibe 2009). Smoking tobacco is a very bad idea for any dancer, but particularly harmful for any dancer with a history of asthma. Dancers who persist in the use of tobacco harm themselves as well as those around them with the passive smoke that they leave behind.

E-cigarettes as a tobacco alternative

We have all seen them—the smoking refugees, standing in a huddled mass outside a building, freezing, getting one last hit before going in to dance. E-cigarettes are marketed as a safe and smokeless way to get a nicotine fix. These electronic cigarettes deliver nicotine to your lung in doses that are supposed to be smaller than standard cigarettes. E-cigarettes themselves, however, may be addictive. Whether or not e-cigarettes will be a helpful alternative that may allow some smokers to transition away from real cigarettes remains a question without a firm answer.

The marketing of e-cigarettes could possibly confuse some dancers into thinking that these electronic cigarettes are a safe alternative to smoking tobacco cigarettes and not a device to be used to attempt to quit smoking. There is absolutely no assurance that this is in fact the case. The Food and Drug Administration found in their preliminary investigation that certain e-cigarettes, just like regular cigarettes, delivered harmful substances such as diethylene glycol to your lungs. It remains controversial how safe ee-cigarettes are to use and the FDA is considering banning their use in the United States.

DANCE CLASS AND YOUR HEART

Dance class—you know how it is: the music starts. Everyone dances for a minute and then the teacher stops the music and corrects everyone! Dance is fabulous for creating long, strong, lean muscles. Dance is excellent for training balance and speed of movement. Dance is not fantastic as a cardiac exercise program.

Your heart is a very important muscle (Fig. 4-2).

To exercise your heart, you need to exercise in a way that really makes that heart muscle work at or near its maximal rate. Dance usually will not do this because the dance sequences are usually too brief. Contrary to many dancers' belief, ballet class is not a complete conditioning program.

The type of exercise called *cardiovascular exercise* is what gets your heart in better condition. To condition your heart, it needs regular exercise, just like the class you take to get your leg and torso muscles ready for dance. Ideally, you would do cardiovascular exercise like swimming, rowing, cross-country skiing, biking, or treadmill for approximately thirty minutes at least four times weekly. The Centers for

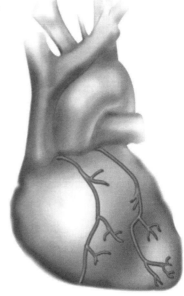

FIG 4-2

Disease Control recommends using 1000 calories a week in exercise. If you walk a half hour daily at a moderate pace for one week, you have used more than your 1000 calories. Most people should be able to fit this amount of cardiovascular exercise into their weekly schedule. We will discuss conditioning and dance in greater detail in Chapter 10.

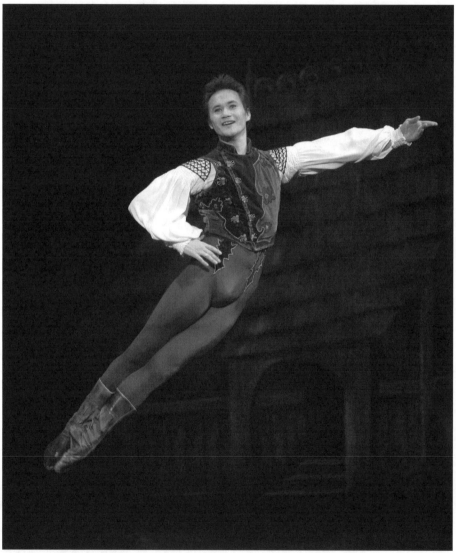

PENNSYLVANIA BALLET PRINCIPAL DANCER ALEXANDER IZILIAEV IN BEN STEVENSON'S *DRACULA*. PHOTOGRAPH BY PAUL KOLNIK.

Five Heart-Lung Issues for Dancers

1. Even thirty hours of dance a week do not constitute a cardiovascular conditioning program. Dancers need to exercise their heart muscle as well as their leg muscles.

2. If your chest gets tight or you are short of breath after exercising, you might have exercise-induced asthma and you need to talk with your doctor about getting checked for this condition. If you have asthma and you also have shortness of breath predictably provoked by exercising, you also need to talk with your doctor to see if your asthma medication needs to be changed to give you better control.

3. You can help control asthma attacks by turning up the studio heat, humidifying the air, and keeping the dance area dust, pet, smoke, and smog free.

4. Smoking cigarettes as a way to control weight is a terrible idea.

5. E-cigarettes may be a way to help break a smoking addiction, but they should not be thought of as a perfectly safe and harmless habit. The safety data are simply not yet available.

Five Lung Exercises for Dancers

1. Blow up balloons—simple and effective.

2. Inhale deeply, slowly let out the air. Repeat ten times daily.

3. Deep breathing awareness: relax. Put both hands on your stomach. Breathe through your nose. Feel how the breaths move your thorax. You could place your hands on your ribs and feel their movement as you do this exercise. Exhale through your mouth. Repeat this exercise and number 4 for about 5–10 minutes (Davis et al. 2008, 1982, 38).

4. Natural breathing: you should inhale through your nose, filling your lower lung, then middle lung, then upper lung. When our attention is tremendously focused our rhythm of breathing can be affected. Deeper breaths can help with muscle relaxation (Davis et al. 2008, 1982, 35, 37-38).

5. Endurance exercise: moderate walking, biking, hiking, elliptical machine—each of these improves heart and lung function and will help your lung capacity.

References

Anawalt, Sasha. 1996. *The Joffrey Ballet: Robert Joffrey and the Making of an American Dance Company*. Chicago, IL: University of Chicago Press.

Curado, Maria Paula and Mia Hashibe. 2009. "Recent Changes in the Epidemiology of Head and Neck Cancer." *Opinion in Oncology* 21 (3, May): 194–200.

Davis, Martha, Elizabeth Robbins Eshelmann, and Matthew McKay, and Patrick Fanning. 2008, 1982. *The Relaxation and Stress Reduction Workbook*, second, sixth edition. Oakland, CA: New Harbinger Publications.

Micheli, Lylref and Mark Jenkins. 2001. *The Sports Medicine Bible for Young Athletes*. Naperville, IL: Sourcebooks, Inc.

Morgan, Christina. 2009. "The E-Cigarette: A Bad Moon Rising?" *The Pump Handle: The Water Cooler for the Public Health Crowd*. June 5. http://thepumphandle.wordpress.com/2009/06/05/e-cigarettes/.

Moss, Dena Simon and Allison Kyle Leopold. 1999. *The Joffrey Ballet School's Ballet-Fit*. New York: St. Martin's Press.

Oreb, Goran, Lana Ruzić, Branka Matković, Marjeta Misigoj-Duraković, Jadranka Vlasić, and Dubravka Ciliga. 2006. "Physical Fitness, Menstrual Cycle Disorders and Smoking Habit in Croatian National Ballet and National Folk Dance Ensembles." *Collegium Antropologicum* 30 (2, June): 279–283.

Pumariega, Andres, Leonardo Rodriguez, and Mark Kilgus. 2004. "Substance Abuse among Adolescents: Current Perspectives." *Addictive Disorders and Their Treatment*. 3 (4, December): 145-155.

U.S. Department of Health and Human Services. 2006. *The Surgeon General's Call to Action to Prevent and Decrease Overweight and Obesity*. Rockville, MD: U.S. Department of Health and Human Services, Public Health Service, Office of the Surgeon General.

———. 2010. *The Surgeon General's Vision for a Healthy and Fit Nation*. Rockville, MD: U.S. Department of Health and Human Services, Office of the Surgeon General (January).

Werner, Mark J., Susan L. Rosenthal, and Frank M. Biro. 1991. "Medical Needs of Performing Arts Students." *Journal of Adolescent Health* 12 (4, June): 294–300.

Wikipedia, s.v. "Asthma," http://en.wikipedia.org/wiki/Asthma.

Zezima, Katie. 2009. "Cigarettes Without Smoke, or Regulation." *The New York Times* June 1, 2nd edition in print: A1.

5 The Importance of Diet

What is a diet?

MOST OF US THINK OF A DIET AS WHAT WE *DO NOT* EAT. "HEY, I'M ON A DIET!" THAT TRANSLATES INTO, "HEY! I'M DEPRIVING MYSELF. I AM NOT EATING NOW WHAT I WOULD NORMALLY EAT." THIS IS NOT A GOOD WAY TO THINK ABOUT A DIET!

A diet is what we *should* normally eat to serve as fuel for our bodies. This nutritional fuel is used so that we can grow appropriately, so that we can heal from injury, and so that we may be able to reproduce. When we do *not* eat a diet that gives us adequate nutrition, we take longer to heal from injuries; we get stress fractures; we experience fatigue; and we lose the ability to reproduce because the menstrual cycle either shuts itself down—a condition called *amenorrhea*—or never starts up until after you are 16 years old—a condition called *primary amenorrhea*.

Why is it important to have a diet that includes all essential nutrients?

Nutrition is not something you can think about once a season, as in, "Well *Nutcracker* is done, so now I can eat! I am going to polish off an entire turkey and a whole apple pie." Dancers who skip class all week and then try to make it all up with one marathon run at the choreography either get nowhere or, even worse, injure themselves. *Similarly, with nutrition, if you deprive yourself of proper nutrition for the majority of the season—or for your entire career on stage—you may cause permanent damage to your body.* You will have less energy and more injuries. It is very important that all dancers pay attention to getting adequate nutrition through their daily diet.

Why ballet dancers often have a disordered diet

The sleek look of ballet means that dancers are under pressure to keep their body weight low. Some studies show that dancers aim for a body weight that is 82% of the ideal body weight for their height (Stretanski and Weber 2002, 384). Dancers have a much lower percentage body fat than all but the ultra-elite athletes. Many experts believe that the amount of control and discipline necessary to dance professionally can have a negative impact on control issues related to the diet, leading to an increased risk of dietary deprivation. The pressure of the mirror, the pressure of the competition with other dancers for attention and casting, and the pressure from the teacher—all add up to exact a toll on both male and female dancers.

In 2009 at the International Association for Dance Medicine and Science (IADMS) meeting, a researcher presented data on how the mirror affected the performances of the dance students at her academy. Based on ease of movement, accuracy, and alignment, Sally Radell and her colleagues found that the higher-level dancers felt more positive about body image when they did not train with a mirror (Radell, Adame, and Cole 2009). Periods of time training without the use of a mirror may be a good idea for higher-level students to become more comfortable with body image.

The female athletic triad

The female dancer faces some unique challenges. Irregular periods occur in more than 60% of female dancers compared to approximately 5% irregular periods in a non-athletic population (Holschen 2004, 853). The female athletic triad is diagnosed when the following occur: 1. disordered eating, 2. altered menstrual function, and 3. decreased ability to lay down normal amounts of bone (IADMS Education Committee 2000). The female athletic triad is found more commonly in all sports where low body mass is a competitive advantage. There is no sport, however, that practices the majority of the time in front of a mirror (in spandex) as dance does!

EATING DISORDERS

Eating disorders defined

Anorexia nervosa: when the person's weight is less than 85% of expected body weight, that is self imposed, with a distorted body image, and the absence of three consecutive menstrual periods. Anorexia nervosa is a very serious medical condition that can be fatal.

Bulimia nervosa: bulimia is a disease of binging. If you are binging on foods and then performing hours and hours of exercise, or inducing vomiting after the binge, you have the hallmarks of bulimia nervosa. People with bulimia characteristically experience intense food cravings. There is a cycle—crave, binge, and exercise or purge.

Eating disorder not otherwise specified: weight loss but not yet less than 85% of expected body weight. Women may have only missed a period or two. They may binge or they may purge but they do not binge and purge in the cycle we described above (The Renfrew Center Foundation; LeBrun in Maffulli et al).

The risk factors

Athletes generally, and dancers in particular, are at high risk of developing an eating disorder. Female dance students are at much higher risk than male dance students for having an eating disorder. Dancers who are chronically "dieting" are probably at a higher risk for an eating disorder. Those who compulsively exercise, explaining, "I ate an extra French fry and now I am going to have to run a mile," are at risk for eating disorders. The dancer who literally cannot stop or slow down—who does not sleep, who has general hyperactivity all the time, who dances all day and then goes for a run at night—can be at increased risk for an eating disorder. The dancer who does not have a positive self-image and who is destructively self-critical, who truly feels that she or he never gets it right, always has a terrible class, always feels fat, and frequently asks others to confirm his or her negative concept of themselves are at risk for eating disorders. "Did you see how off that pirouette was? I look really fat today!" These are all warning signs that a dancer may be at risk of having or developing an eating disorder.

Dancers who think they may have an eating disorder should talk to a medical doctor and get help. The Renfrew Center is a medical care center devoted to the treatment of eating disorders with a website packed with helpful information. Check out the website at www.renfrewcenter.com.

Dancers at risk for eating disorders

Preprofessional companies and conservatories are trying to become more aware of potential problems with screening questions—but most dancers simply overstate their caloric intake and may be less than forthright about their menstrual cycle. This silence of dancers' not reporting accurately about eating habits, diet, and daily food intake is hard to break. The absence of menstrual cycles in a dancer should be considered a significant potential problem and should not be assumed to be benign and without consequence (Warren 1999). Even dancers who do not meet all the criteria for anorexia nervosa may have an eating disorder.

HEALTHY BONES, HEALTHY DANCER

How can I help my bone health?

The International Association for Dance Medicine and Science (IADMS) has issued some helpful advice in a paper called "Bone Health and Female Dancers: Physical and Nutritional Guidelines" (Robson and Chertoff 2008). You need sufficient calcium in your diet; if you do not get enough calcium, your body starts stealing what it needs from your bones. This is not a good thing!

The National Institutes of Health (NIH) recommend that everyone fourteen to eighteen years old gets 1,300 mg. of calcium intake a day; that those nineteen to fifty years old have an intake of 1,000 mg. of calcium daily; and those over fifty have a daily intake of 1,200 mg. of calcium. (Separate NIH intake guidelines are recommended for those who are pregnant or breast-feeding.)

Vitamin D, naturally available from sunlight and certain foods, causes calcium to be absorbed. Long studio hours of dance and fluorescent lights do not help your body get adequate vitamin D. Get your 15 minutes a day in the sun for adequate vitamin D. Dairy products such as yogurt and cheese are another good source of vitamin D. Dancers who do not get enough calcium through their regular diet should consider taking calcium supplements to reach approximately 1000–1200 mg. of calcium intake daily. Vitamin D 800 IU is often included in calcium supplements. Also, some calcium supplements are chewable for those who just cannot swallow a pill.

We create most of our future bone density by age twenty. In the female athlete, reduced energy availability—not enough food to meet your need—is probably the number one culprit causing athletic amenorrhea (the absence of menstruation secondary to exercise). So if you eat enough calories, you help protect your bones.

Some dancers get placed on oral contraceptives in an effort to increase bone mass. One group of researchers even studied alendronate (Fosamax®) for the treatment of decreased bone mass in patients with anorexia nervosa (Golden et al. 2005, 3183-3184). Alendronate stops your body from leaching calcium from bone that is already laid down in your skeleton. Basically, alendronate slows the resorption of bone and is usually used to treat postmenopausal women with low bone mass. Even a strong medicine like a biphosphonate such as Fosamax® was less effective than increasing caloric intake and weight in having a positive effect on bone mass. Also the biphosphonates can cause other health issues such as rashes and jaw problems. The use of biphosphonates by the dancer who is still growing remains questionable because of unanswered safety questions. Hormone replacement therapy also was not as successful as increasing nutritional intake.

Because dancers are at risk for eating disorders and for osteoporosis, and because we know they may not accurately report their periods, perhaps dancers should get bone density studies at age 15 and then again at age 16. We would know then if they are having problems laying down adequate bone and at least would have the potential to get treated or to increase dietary intake.

Osteoporosis

Osteoporosis, a condition in which the bone is weaker than normal, has been studied in ballet dancers (Warren 1999; Nemet and Eliakim 2009; Robson and Chertoff 2008). Dancers sometimes get stress fractures, which are different from fractures such as breaking your leg from an acute trauma like falling off a horse. A stress fracture can happen just because you dance too much and overstress the bone. Then the bone cannot heal quickly enough from the stress, and the bone fractures.

Dancers with too little bone mass or osteoporosis are at increased risk for having more problems with stress fractures. Late onset of the first period (after age 16), menstrual cycle irregularity, low calcium intake, long hours of training—all are risk factors for developing osteoporosis. To some degree, weight-bearing exercise can help with bone health. But if a dancer has disordered menstrual cycles, this protective effect of exercise is not sufficient to prevent the development of stress fractures. Lower serum estrogen is the key. That means that if you are not menstruating normally you are at a high risk for weaker bones and stress fractures. Calcium intake, alcohol intake, and even cigarette smoking seem to be less important risk factors for having a problem with your bone health than abnormal menses.

DIETARY SUPPLEMENTS

Carbohydrates: Energy drinks are loaded with carbohydrates. Most of these drinks contain approximately 60-80 gram/liter of carbohydrates, most commonly glucose. Carbohydrate content might be listed: 60-80 gram/liter would be listed as approximately 6–8% carbohydrates (Juekendroup, ed. 214). The ingredients in energy drinks are water, sugar, caffeine, and numerous supplements. Most energy drinks have plenty of calories so check that label and compare your sports drink to good old orange juice. Read the label on your energy drink! There is little documentation to support the use of these drinks.

Most dancers probably need a diet of about 50% carbohydrates. The IADMS Nutrition Fact Sheet suggests that dancers eat complex carbohydrates such as cereal, bread, pastas, and muffins—not simple sugars. Simple sugars such as table sugar generally do not provide additional nutrition and are low in fiber (Clarkson 2003–2005).

Protein: Most adults need about 12% of their diet from proteins, which are the building blocks of muscles. Proteins help us heal, provide energy for performance, and they are important to nerve function. Because muscles and nerves provide the power and control of movement in dance, inadequate protein intake will affect your dance performance capabilities and your ability to recover from injury.

Your protein intake ideally would be approximately 1.4–1.6 gram of protein per kg. of body weight per day. A 50 kg. dancer weighing approximately 110 pounds would therefore require approximately 75 grams of protein or 2.65 ounces. (IADMS Nutrition Fact Sheet—Fueling the Dancer). Some simple ways to increase protein in your diet is through whey and soy powders that can be placed into smoothies or other foods.

Creatine: Creatine supplements build muscle mass and improve performance in activities that require high-energy outputs. The male dancer is probably the most likely to use creatine, yet no one knows how safe creatine is for young athletes. Creatine supplementation may be associated with weight gain, muscle cramps, and complaints of nausea and diarrhea. So dancer beware! (Jeukendroup and Gleeson 2010, 275–281).

Carnitine: although carnitine helps with building bone mass, oral carnitine probably will not help with loss of muscle fat. It also probably does not really work as a weight loss agent. It seems that our bodies tightly regulate the enzymes that are involved in the carnitine pathway and help it to function at a maximum level anyway. Therefore, it is unlikely that supplementation help the majority of dancers.

Caffeine: Caffeine is a stimulant. Shakes, racing heart, and the jitters can all be an effect of caffeine. Watch the ingredient list carefully of your high-energy drink to make sure that you do not shake on stage!

Fluids: Most adults go through about 8 – 12 cups a day of fluids. Assuming that you sweat about four cups a day (at least!) in dance class, you need to make sure you adjust your fluid intake accordingly. Do not be the plant wilting in the sun from too-low fluids. Too-low fluid intake leads to fatigue and weakness. Too-low fluid intake in a hot studio leads to heat exhaustion! Some symptoms of heat exhaustion include nausea, dizziness, bad muscle cramping, rapid heart rate, fainting, and even disorientation. Heat exhaustion means that your body simply cannot get cool enough through sweating. If you start to feel any of the above symptoms you need to stop your activity, get to a cool room, and drink cool fluids.

Heat exhaustion can progress and be very serious. Any dancer with severe symptoms of heat exhaustion or symptoms that persist more than about one hour should seek medical care. In fact, dancers with any dizziness, nausea, very hot skin, or rapid pulse need to seek immediate medical attention because these symptoms may be a warning sign of the medical emergency called *heat stroke.*

Iron: iron allows your blood cells to carry oxygen properly and this oxygen allows your muscles to work correctly. Probably 25–50% of athletes are iron deficient (anemic). Most athletes, and in particular female athletes, do not get enough iron in their diets. Doctors who rely on serum ferritin as a measure of your iron stores may be misled by levels that may be falsely elevated in dancers because of the intense exercise they do in dance class. Their more-than-thirty hours a week may cause an artificial bump in the ferritin from inflammation associated with that exercise (Nemet and Eliakim 2009).

It is important to note that anemia in dancers is a condition that may have a very slow onset. Because of this, your body may get used to being anemic and you might not realize that you have this medical problem. It is important to know whether or not you are anemic because of the short-term impact of anemia on your energy levels and the long-term effect of anemia on your health. So get yourself checked by your doctor at your regular physical if you are a dancer to make sure that you and your blood iron levels are OK.

THE VEGETARIAN DANCER

Vegetarian dancers need to be careful that their protein needs are being met adequately by their diet. Plant proteins are digested differently than animal protein. An increase in protein intake of 10% compared to the usual recommended amount is a good idea. As a result, vegetarian athletes are at relatively high risk of iron deficiency. Vegetarian athletes can help themselves by eating iron-fortified breakfast cereals and green, leafy vegetables with a high iron content. Proper amounts of fat intake, B12, riboflavin, vitamin D, and calcium are also issues for vegetarians. All dancers who have restricted diets should have periodic monitoring by a physician or nutritionist to make sure their dietary requirements are being met.

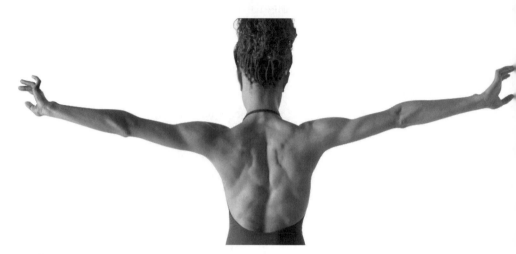

FORMER PENNSYLVANIA BALLET COMPANY MEMBER HEIDI CRUZ. PHOTOGRAPH BY STEVE BELKOWITZ.

Five Key Things to Know about Nutrition

1. Not getting enough calories causes menstrual dysfunction and loss of muscle and bone. Your daily diet needs to be able to support your body's activities! If you are restricting a food group, you still need to get the necessary nutrients of that food group or there will be a negative impact on your health.

2. Dancers need to be sure to get adequate calcium so they do not develop problems with their bone mass.

3. Vitamin D is essential so that you can absorb calcium. The American Academy of Pediatrics recommends 400 IU of vitamin D intake daily in teenagers. The NIH suggests a value of 600 IU of vitamin D intake daily in teenagers and those nineteen-to-fifty years old. Some people will need to use supplements to get adequate vitamin D intake.

4. Dehydration is common and causes fatigue and decreased muscle power. If you are a dancer who is constantly getting cramps after performance you may need to allow yourself more fluids and sodium. Remember to hydrate before, during, and after dance.

5. Vegetarian dancers are at higher risk of nutritional deficiency. You should probably get checked by a doctor periodically to see that your body has enough iron and other nutrients.

Five Key Ingredients for the Dancer's Diet

1. Carbohydrates are optimally about 50– 65% of a dancer's diet.

2. Fats are optimally 20–25% of a dancer's diet.

3. Protein builds muscle; 12–15 % of the dancer's diet should be protein.

4. Five servings of fruit and vegetables a day should be part of your daily intake.

5. Hydration matters. Fluids, fluids, fluids! Dancers who drink more have less hunger and have less fatigue.

References

American Dietetic Association and Dietitians of Canada. "Nutrition and Athletic Performance—Joint Position Paper." American College of Sports Medicine. *Medicine and Science in Sports and Exercise* 41, no. 3 (2009): 709–731.

Clarkson, Priscilla. "Nutrition Fact Sheet: Fueling the Dancer." *International Association for Dance Medicine and Science* (2003, 2005): 1–2.

Golden, Neville H. "Eating disorders in Adolescence: What is the Role of Hormone Replacement Therapy?" *Current Opinion in Obstetrics and Gynecology* 19, no. 5 (October 2007): 434–439.

Golden N. H, E. A. Iglesias, M. S. Jacobson, D. Carey, W. Meyer , J. Schebendach, S. Hertz, and I. R. Shenker. "Alendronate for the Treatment of Osteopenia in Anorexia Nervosa: A Randomized, Double-Blind, Placebo-Controlled Trial." *Journal of Clinical Endocrinology and Metabolism* 90, no. 6 (2005): 3179–3185.

Holschen, Jolie C. "The Female Athlete." *Southern Medical Journal* 97, no. 9 (September 2004): 852–858.

IADMS Education Committee. "The Challenge of the Adolescent Dancer." *International Association for Dance Medicine and Science* (2001).

Jeukendrup, Asker and Michael Gleeson Michael. 2010. *Sport Nutrition: An Introduction to Energy Production and Performance,* 2nd edition. Champaign, IL: Human Kinetics.

Kilicarslan, Alpaslan, Mehlika Isildak, Gulay Sain Guven, S. Gul Oz, Aylin Hasbay, Erdem Karablut, and Tumay Sozen. "The Influence of Ballet Training on Bone Mass in Turkish Ballet Dancers." *The Endocrinologist* 17, no. 2 (March/April 2007): 85–88.

LeBrun, Constance M. "Female Athletic Triad." In *Sports Medicine for Specific Ages and Abilities,* edited by Nicola Maffulli, Kai Ming Chan, Rose Macdonald, Robert A. Malina, and Anthony W. Parker. London, UK: Churchill Livingstone, 2001.

Nemet, Dan and Alon Eliakim. "Pediatric Sports Nutrition: An Update." *Current Opinion in Clinical Nutrition and Metabolic Care* 12, no. 3 (May 2009): 304–309.

Office of Dietary Supplements, National Institutes of Health. "Dietary Supplement Fact Sheet: Calcium." Last update October 2009. http://ods.od.nih.gov/factsheets/Calcium_pf.asp.

——"Dietary Supplement Fact Sheet: Vitamin D. Health Professional Fact Sheet." Last update 13 November, 2009. http://ods.od.nih.gov/factsheets/vitamind.asp.

"Dietary Supplement Fact Sheet: Vitamin D Consumer." Last update 30 November, 2010. http://ods.od.nih.gov/FactSheets/VitaminD-Consumer/

Radell, Sally A., Daniel D. Adame and Steven P. Cole. "The Impact of Mirrors on Body Image in High and Low Performing Female Ballet Students." Presentation at the International Association for Dance Medicine and Science, 19th annual meeting. The Hague, The Netherlands, October 30, 2009.

Renfrew Center Foundation. "Eating Disorders Signs and Symptoms." *Renfrew Educational Materials.* http://renfrew.org/resources/documents/Eating_Disorders_Signs_and_Symptoms.pdf

Robson, Bonnie and Arlene Chertoff. 2008. "Bone Health and Female Dancers: Physical and Nutritional Guidelines." *International Association for Dance Medicine and Science.*

Shah, Selina. "Iron Deficiency: Diagnosis, Effects, and Management." Presentation at the International Association for Dance Medicine and Science, 19th annual meeting. The Hague, The Netherlands, October 30, 2009.

Stretanski, M. F. and G. J. Weber. "Medical and Rehabilitation Issues in Classical Ballet: Literature Review." *American Journal of Physical Medicine and Rehabilitation* 81 (2002): 383–391.

6 The Low Back or Lumbar Spine

ANATOMY: THE FUNCTIONAL UNIT AND HOW IT WORKS

YOUR LOW BACK WORKS WHEN YOU TWIST, LIFT, JUMP, BEND, AND EXTEND IT (FIG. 6-1). THE MOVEMENT LOOKS EFFORTLESS. BUT SMALL AND LARGE LOW BACK MUSCLES ARE WORKING AWAY TO ALLOW THESE MOVEMENTS TO OCCUR. TO ACCOMPLISH THESE ASTONISHING FEATS, YOUR SPINE IS LINKED INTO FUNCTIONAL UNITS.

Each functional unit of your spine includes the following: two back bones called *lumbar vertebrae* linked together by a disc in between, the small facet joints of the vertebrae that connect the vertebral bones as they combine into a joint toward the back of the vertebra, the arches behind the vertebral bodies, and the ligaments and muscles that help tie everything together (Fig. 6-2).

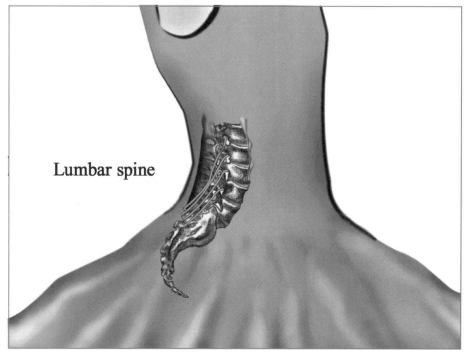

Lumbar spine

FIG 6-1

FIG 6-2

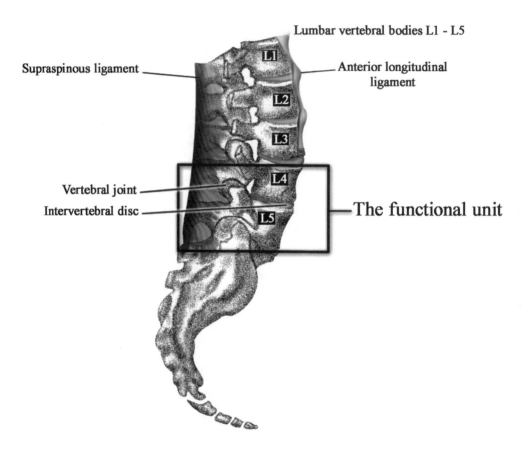

Lumbar vertebral bodies L1 - L5

Supraspinous ligament

Anterior longitudinal ligament

L1

L2

L3

L4

L5

Vertebral joint

Intervertebral disc

The functional unit

The detailed anatomy of what makes up a functional unit of the lumbar spine is less important for you to understand than the concept behind how a functional unit works—that forces get coordinated by the structures between two lumbar vertebrae and the bones themselves rather than impinging upon one individual area. The functional units thus absorb force, allow motion, and protect nerves (Nordin and Frankel 2001, 256–258).

The vertebral bodies

The front of the functional unit of each vertebra is called the *vertebral body*. It is a solid bone cylinder designed to carry your weight. Part of the reason bone density from consuming calcium is important is that the lack of enough bone strength translates into a higher risk of fracture in weight-bearing structures like the spine. A spine that has vertebral bodies that look like Swiss cheese will tend to get tiny fractures with the loading of dance movements and landing from high leaps. *Osteopenia* is the technical term for low bone mass density that is not too severe. Osteoporosis is defined by even more severe loss of bone (Fig. 6-3). (See Chapter 5 for additional information about osteoporosis.)

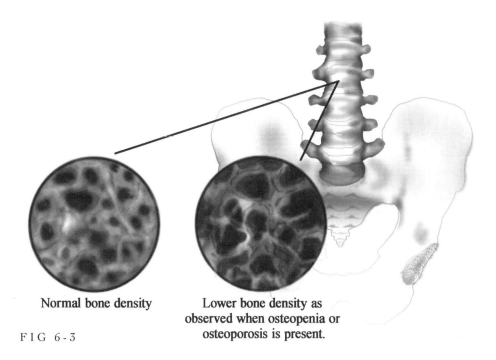

Normal bone density

Lower bone density as observed when osteopenia or osteoporosis is present.

FIG 6-3

The intervertebral discs

Between each two lumbar vertebral bodies is a lumbar disc. The disc is often described as a jelly doughnut because it has a soft center and an outer fibrous ring. Jelly doughnuts are probably not helpful images for dancers, however, so we will talk about it as a belt surrounding a glob of absorbing gel (Fig. 6-4).

Lumbar disc

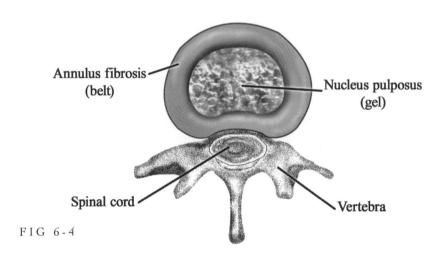

Annulus fibrosis
(belt)

Nucleus pulposus
(gel)

Spinal cord

Vertebra

FIG 6-4

The gel can rebound from twisting, compression, stretching, and bending. However, if the outer strap is twisted too much, or the forces on the gel become too great, the strap can tear, allowing the gel to escape, or the gel pack can shoot against the belt strap causing it to bulge (Fig. 6-5).

Herniated lumbar disc

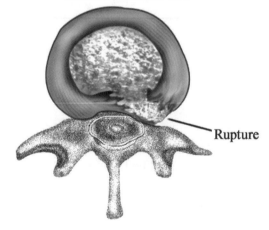

Rupture

FIG 6-5

As you age, there is less water in the gel cushion in the disc and so the ability of the disc to sustain pressure loads decreases. In addition, you will become tighter and tighter as your available spine motion decreases. Your available motion drops by approximately 30% for lumbar range of motion from youth to the time you are about seventy years of age (Nordin and Frankel 2001, 263–264). This is partly why we do not see 75-year-old prima ballerinas performing on stage. Your body, quite literally, will not have the necessary range of motion.

In the normal population—that is, non-dancers—the loss in lumbar range of motion is usually compensated for by increased hip motion (Nordic and Frankel 2001, 264). Dancers simply cannot do this because it is likely that they have been using all their available hip range of motion their entire careers. As a result, no room exists for compensation from hip motion to make up for the lack of spine mobility.

As the discs lose their hydration and elasticity with aging, there is also more impact on the vertebral bodies. The vertebral bodies then start to show signs of degeneration, developing arthritic spikes and spurs, which can crowd the available central space where the big bundle of lumbosacral nerves are located (Fig. 6-6).

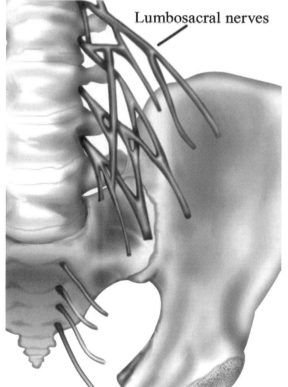

Lumbosacral nerves

When the space for the nerves is too tight, dancers can develop chronic irritation in these nerves that causes tingling, numbness, and leg pain. There can be chronic low back pain. This condition is called *spinal stenosis*. Degenerative spinal stenosis is generally a condition of the older dancer since the spurs

FIG 6-6

take time to develop. However, some younger dancers may have problems with lumbar stenosis causing low back pain because they were born with a relatively narrow space for the nerves. This is called *congenital* (from birth) *stenosis* as opposed to *degenerative stenosis*. Any dancer with pain down both legs needs to be checked for congenital spinal stenosis.

The functional unit posterior

The vertebral bodies have two thick processes that protrude off the back called *pedicles* that connect in turn to two laminas to form a protected space for the horsehair tail of your spinal nerves. The pedicles and laminas together make up the vertebral arch. The solid vertebral body that carries the majority of your weight is therefore in front of a hollow vertebral arch.

The facet joints are a series of overlapping plates that keep your spine stable and help distribute weight. The lumbar facet joints are particularly stressed in extension. Arabesque, for example, will preferentially shift loads onto the lumbar facets and can irritate the lumbar facet joints quite a bit.

Dancers who do not control arabesque well, or who have weak abdominal muscles, can stress the pedicles and develop what is called a *pars fracture* (see page 71).

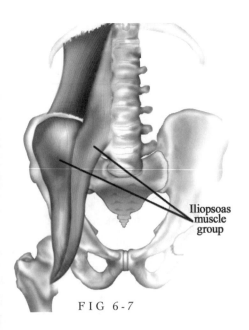

Iliopsoas muscle group

FIG 6-7

SPINE ANATOMY—MUSCLES

You bend forward and backward and side to side. Spine flexion, extension, and lateral or side flexion are accomplished by the contraction of muscles moving functional spine units. The muscles in front of your spine are your abdominal muscles and your iliopsoas. Generally speaking, these muscles flex your spine (Fig. 6-7).

Behind your spine are the back extensor muscles. The erector spinae, multifidus, and intertransversarii muscles, generally speaking, extend your spine.

If you contract asymmetrically—for example if you use your right abdominal flexors and your left lumbar extensors—your spine will tend to twist. Additionally, there are spine rotational muscles that assist with twisting your spine. If your muscles are fatigued, extra stress gets placed on the passive bony and ligamentous structures of your spine, making you a setup for injury and low back pain.

On the other hand, you need to be careful in how you exercise to increase lumbar and abdominal muscle strength. The exercises that you do should not cause extra stress on your low back. One simple modification in strengthening your abdominal muscles, for example, is to substitute a limited curl-up exercise for a regular curl-up. Keep your knees bent and limit your curl-up to just clearing your shoulder blades. Keep your back flat on the floor. This limited curl-up remains effective in building abdominal muscle strength but is less stressful to the spine (Fig. 6.8). Also, a reverse curl, bringing your hips off the floor, is an effective exercise that puts less stress on your spine (Nordin and Frankel 2001, 276–277).

**Limited curl-up technique
keeping the back flat on the floor**

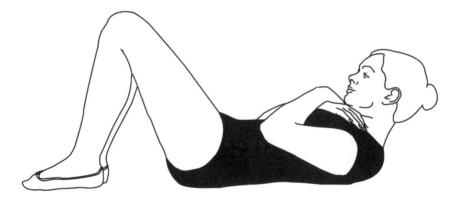

FIG 6-8

SPINE ANATOMY—NERVES

The nerves in your low back are in a horsehair brush called the *cauda equina*. This brush separates into individual spinal nerve roots. The spine roots combine to form nerves that provide sensation and cue the muscles in your legs. A disc bulge or a disc herniation in your low back means that a part of the disc pillow that normally sits between two vertebral bones has moved out of place. Sometimes this happens from a twisting injury that tears part of the belt that keeps the disc in place or from a sudden heavy lift. A disc can press against the spine roots because of this disc bulge, or herniation, causing pain.

LOW BACK PAIN IN DANCE

Low back pain is very common in dancers. Doctors Shah and Weiss surveyed modern dancers and found that the low back injury occurs almost as often as the ankle injury—17.4% low back injuries compared to 17.8% ankle injuries (Shah and Weiss 2006, 437). It is very important for dancers to know what types of low back pain should cause them to get immediate medical attention. These are called "red flags" because they may indicate a more serious problem than just a low back muscle being pulled and causing pain.

The red flags of low back pain in dance

1. Your partner had you in an overhead lift and dropped you on the floor and you have pain.

2. Your partner was doing pirouettes and kicked you in the back and you have pain.

3. Your diet is terrible, your calcium intake is negligible, and/or you smoke—and you have low back pain.

4. You have been treated for any type of cancer and now you have low back pain.

5. You have fever, chills, and back pain.

6. You have weight loss and you have low back pain

7. You have had a recent infection, even if it is a urinary tract infection or what you thought was a minor skin infection or cold, and now you have low back pain.

8. You have recently been taking steroids or any drug that might decrease your immune function—and you have low back pain.

9. You have low back pain that is worse when you lie down at night.

10. Your back pain persists even when you are not dancing.

11. You have had low back pain for more than two weeks.

12. Your pain is severe.

13. Your leg is weak, painful, or numb.

14. You have any change in your bladder or bowel function.

15. You are older than 50 or younger than 20 years old and you have low back pain.

16. You do not have normal menstrual periods and you have low back pain.

It is very true that most low back pain is troubling but transient and is gone in less than four weeks. But it is also true that some of the most lingering injuries in dance are injuries to the low back. Generally speaking, most dancers with low back pain should be checked by their physician before beginning their rehabilitation program.

Lumbar strain in dance muscle and ligament injury

Dancers with lumbar strains often have pain in the mid-back or the muscles to the side of the spine. Overusing the muscles will cause pain and low back stiffness. This pain should not become chronic. Lumbar strains do not cause radiating pain into the leg typically and an acute twisting strain or overuse strain should start feeling better pretty quickly—within a day or two. Stretching your hamstrings and applying ice or heat will help.

It is important to keep your back muscles strong. When dancers have back fatigue but continue to do lifts, they increase the risk straining their muscles as well as injuring the other structures of their backs, such as the discs, nerves, and facets (Kong, et al. 1996).

Facet joint pain

The repeated hyperextensions (bending your lumbar spine backwards beyond what is your normal range of motion) of dance can cause the facet joints to jam up against each other and bruise each other (Trepman, Walaszek, and Micheli 2005, 91). Facet joint pain is often more localized than a lumbar strain of the muscles. It is usually on one side of your back as opposed to low back strains that spread across your back.

If you have persistent facet joint pain, direct spine mobilization techniques by a manual physical therapist or chiropractor will take the stress off the joint. You can then begin a rehabilitation program. If physical therapy, exercise, and manual therapy do not correct your problem your doctor and you could consider a referral to a medical specialist for anesthetic medial branch blocks of the nerves to the facet joints or possible facet joint injections. Both medial branch blocks and facet joint injections are only part of a comprehensive approach to managing back pain and need to be incorporated into a comprehensive rehabilitation approach for persistent low back pain issues in dancers.

Lumbar disc injury in dance

If the gel in the disc bulges out of place, pressure on nerve roots can cause pain that shoots down your leg. This is called radiculopathy or sciatica. Dancers with radiculopathy or sciatica often find that flexing the spine increases their pain. These dancers will also have hamstrings that feel very tight and they may have leg numbness. Rarely, large disc herniations can cause numbness in your buttocks or in what is called the saddle area. Dancers with this type of problem or any loss of bowel or bladder control need emergency evaluation and treatment of what is usually a fairly massive disc herniation. Massive disc herniations that cause this type of saddle numbness or bowel or bladder issues could cause permanent problems if not treated promptly. More commonly, however, dancers with a disc herniation will have low back and pain in one leg.

Aquatic exercise can really help disc pain settle down. Acupuncture can be very effective, too. Finally, epidural steroid injections, which can be done as an outpatient procedure, can help calm down an inflamed nerve root.

Spondylolysis and spondylolisthesis— low back pain with bone injury

Repeated bending and twisting can cause a mechanical fracture of the pars of the lumbar spine of the dancer.

This fracture is called a *spondylolysis*. A pars fracture on one side is bad enough, but if you go on to break the pars on both the right and left then that can cause what is called *spondylolisthesis*, a condition in which the bones actually can slide out of place. A spondylolisthesis can cause chronic low back pain (Fig. 6-9). It is therefore very important to let your spine heal if, in fact, you get a pars fracture, since you certainly do not want to have chronic issues and even potential instability of your spine.

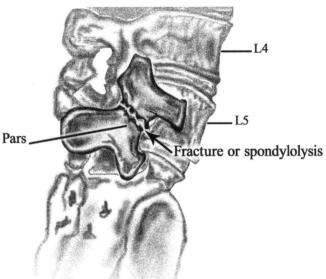

FIG 6-9

In all athletics, these pars fractures of the lumbar spine are more common than you would think; they occur to a great frequency in adolescent dancers with low back pain. The authors Najeeb, Khan, and Haak comment that one study found up to 48% of low back pain in the adolescent athlete is secondary to these fatigue fractures (Najeeb, Khan, and Haak 2008, 22). The pain comes on gradually with significant hamstring tightness and pain in the buttock and back of the thigh. Arabesque will predictably aggravate this pain, as will overhead lifts. Your back will feel really flat and like it is in spasm.

All dancers with continuing low back pain for more than two-to-three weeks should be examined by a medical doctor. They will probably need a two-view lumbar X-Ray scan to evaluate instability or other serious medical issues. Oblique views, however, unnecessarily increase your exposure to radiation and really do not add a great deal of information.

Bone scans and SPECT or "single photon emission computerized tomography scans" will predict if you have a fracture and if it can heal. An active bone scan means there is an active healing process! This is information you need to know.

Approximately 90% of dancers will do well with bracing and allowing the fracture to heal. They need to stop dancing until the fracture has healed. Most dancers can expect to return to dance class in approximately three months. Aquatic exercise is a good rehabilitation program for most dancers with symptomatic spondylolysis because it does not add stress to the spine but still allows you to exercise your muscles.

Lumbar lordosis and ballet

One common problem in ballet dancers is an increased lumbar lordosis, which means that they often increase the arch of the low back. Increasing your back curve increases your apparent turnout, which may be one reason why it is so common. This increased lumbar curve puts extra pressure on your spine and increases your risk of developing low back pain. Eventually, it can lead to a tighter psoas muscle in the front of the thigh. This tight psoas can actually limit the height of leg extensions on that side. Physical therapist Marika Molnar commented on the issue of low extensions in *Pointe* magazine. She recommended Pilates exercises (see below) to help build core strength and abdominal stabilization to treat this type of problem.

MRI as a way to diagnose persistent low back complaints

Dancers and elite athletes put a great deal of stress on lumbar structures. The MRI may show findings that are not necessarily the cause of the dancer's conditions. MRI findings must correlate with your physical exam and the history of your problem. In 2007, a study was done of teenage elite athletes in Britain; asymptomatic tennis players were assessed with lumbar MRI. The findings were really remarkable. Thirteen out of thirty-three players with no symptoms had degenerative disc changes noted on MRI. Twenty-three players out of thirty-three showed abnormalities of the facet joint (Alyas, Turner, and Connell 2007, 837). If you are a dancer with lingering pain, see a dance medicine specialist who can correlate your MRI findings to your exam so you get the correct treatment for the correct problem. Make sure it is YOU and not your MRI that is being treated!

PILATES AND DANCE

Joseph Pilates (1883-1967) created and developed a conditioning program that is immensely popular in dance. He shared a building with New York City Ballet— and the Pilates technique is justly famous for helping keep dancers fit and on stage. The Pilates technique can be very helpful in keeping the spine lengthened and strong. Pilates exercises improve overall flexibility and emphasize core stabilization—excellent for the dancer.

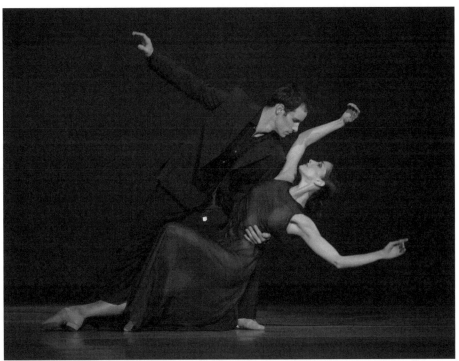

PENNSYLVANIA BALLET PRINCIPAL DANCER RIOLAMA LORENZO AND SOLOIST FRANCIS VEYETTE IN MATTHEW NEENAN'S *PENUMBRA*. PHOTOGRAPH BY PAUL KOLNIK.

Five critical things you need to know
about low back pain in dance

1. Dancers with low back pain for more than two weeks need to be evaluated by a medical professional.

2. Dancers with low back pain and any of the red flags listed earlier in this chapter need to be evaluated by a medical doctor.

3. Spine fatigue fractures are probably under-diagnosed in dance. Because of this, many dancers who might have been able to heal a symptomatic fracture of the spine missed the opportunity and may have set themselves up for future problems. Do not let this be you!

4. MRI is only part of the evaluation of low back pain and may be misleading as to the cause of your symptoms. Doctors treat patients, not MRI scans. Make sure that your doctor is correlating your MRI findings with your symptoms and physical examination findings.

5. Some exercises can be modified so they cause less stress on your spine. Any dancer with a history of low back pain should check with a physical therapist or dance doctor to be certain that his or her spine exercises are being done in a way that minimizes the stress on the low back.

Five great exercises and stretches for dancers

1. Sitting, roll your spine forward and continue into a hamstring stretch. Count for twenty and repeat on other side.

2. Kneel on the floor on all fours. You should be balanced on your knees and extended arms. Lift right arm forward and left leg backward simultaneously and hold for twenty counts. Repeat this exercise 5 to 10 times. Now lift your left arm and right leg simultaneously and repeat the exercise 5 to 10 times.

3. Stand on one leg. Passé your other leg, extend it to the side and hold. Repeat slowly and with good form 5 to 10 times.

4. Stand on one leg. Passé your other leg forward, extend it to the side and hold. Repeat slowly and with good form 5 to 10 times.

5. Lie on your back on the floor with knees bent. Plank with abdominals to lift trunk off the floor. Now do a side plank.

References

Alyas, F., M. Turner and D. Connell. "MRI Findings in the Lumbar Spines of Asymptomatic, Adolescent, Elite Tennis Players." *British Journal of Sports Medicine* 41 (2007): 836–841.

Bryan, Melinda and Suzanne Hawson. "The Benefits of Pilates Exercise in Orthopedic Rehabilitation." *Techniques in Orthopedics* 18, no. 1 (March 2003): 126–129.

Clippinger, Karen Sue. *Dance Anatomy and Kinesiolology.* Champaign, IL: Human Kinetics, 2007: 71–155.

Frino, John, Richard E. McCarthy, Charisse Y. Sparks, and Frances L. McCullough. "Trends in Adolescent Lumbar Disc Herniations." *Spine* 26, no. 5 (September/October, 2006): 579–581.

Fukushima, Rhoda. "Inner Strength: It's Not All in Your Head — Health and Fitness for Life-Core Training ." *Dance* (Dec. 2001): 94–95.

Kong, Wayne Z., Lars G. Gilbertson and James N. Weinstein. "Effects of Muscle Dysfunction on Lumbar Spine Mechanics: A Finite Element Study Based on a Two Motion Segments Mmodel." *Spine* 21, no. 19 (October 1996): 2197–2206.

Magee, David J. *Orthopedic Physical Assessment,* 4th edition. Philadelphia, PA: Saunders, 2002.

McGill, S. M., V. R. Yingling and J. P. Peach. "Three-Dimensional Kinematics and Trunk Muscle Myoelectric Activity in the Elderly Spine — A Database Compared to Young People." *Clinical Biomechanics* 14, no. 6 (July 1999): 389–95.

Najeeb, Khan, Sohail Hussain. and Michael Haak. "Thoracolumbar Injuries in Athletes." *Sports Medicine and Arthroscopy Review* 16, no. 1 (March 2008): 16–25.

Nordin, Margareta and Victor H. Frankel. *Basic Biomechanics of the Musculoskeletal System,* 3rd edition. Baltimore, MD: Lippincott Williams and Wilkins, 2001: 276-277.

Radcliff, Kristen E., Babak S. Kalantar and Charles A. Reitman. "Surgical Management of Spondylolysis and Spondylolisthesis in Athletes: Indications and Return to Play." *Current Sports Medicine Reports* 8, no. 1 (Jan./Feb. 2009): 35-40.

Shah, Selina and David Weiss. "Survey of Injuries Among Professional Modern Dancers: Prevalence, Risk Factors, and Management." Abstracts from the American Medical Society for Sports Medicine Annual Meeting, April 29–May 3, 2006, Miami Beach, FL. *Clinical Journal of Sports Medicine* 16, no. 5 (Sept. 2006): 437.

Trepman, Elly, Arleen Walaszek and Lyle J. Micheli. "Spinal Problems in Dancers." In *Preventing Dance Injuries,* 2nd edition, edited by Ruth Solomon, John Solomon, and Sandra Cerny Minton. Champaign, IL: Human Kinetics, 2005.

Wozny, Nancy. "Cross-Training for Technique ." *Pointe* Magazine (August/September 2009): 50–52.

7 The Hip

HIP ANATOMY: BONE STRUCTURE

YTHE LONG BONE OF YOUR THIGH, THE FEMUR, CONNECTS WITH YOUR PELVIS TO FORM THE HIP JOINT. THE HEAD OF THE FEMUR IS A BALL CALLED--YOU GUESSED RIGHT!--THE *FEMORAL HEAD*. THE BALL OF THE FEMORAL HEAD FITS INTO A SOCKET IN YOUR PELVIC BONE CALLED THE *ACETABULUM*, WHICH IS THE ACTUAL HIP JOINT. JUST REMEMBER, THAT YOUR FEMUR FITS INTO YOUR PELVIS IN A BALL AND SOCKET JOINT.

The pelvic bone where the hip joint is located is also called the *innominate* bone, sometimes called the *os coxae*. The acetabulum, or hip socket, is part of this innominate bone. Finally, the crests at the top of your innominate, or pelvic, bone are the *iliac crests* (Fig. 7-1).

Proper alignment is a key concept in dance. Your teacher will help you determine your proper alignment. If you feel that the tiny bone spikes at the front of your iliac crests are in a straight vertical plane with your pubic bone, you are

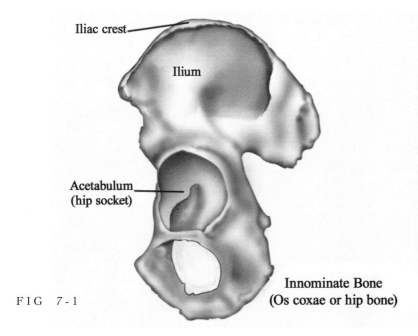

Iliac crest

Ilium

Acetabulum
(hip socket)

Innominate Bone
(Os coxae or hip bone)

FIG   7-1

likely close to a neutral alignment (Deckert 2009, 11). You can tell whether you are tipping your pelvis forward or tucking under in a very simple way: your pubic symphysis is the joint in the midline front of your pelvis that unites the two halves of the pelvic os coxae or innominate bones. Put your fingers at the spiny bumps near the front of your hips. These tiny bumps are the anterior superior iliac spines. Stand and look down at your feet. If your anterior superior iliac spine (ASIS) is in front of your pubic symphysis you are forward tipped at your pelvis. If your ASIS is behind your pubic symphysis you are in a tucked under position (Fig. 7-2).

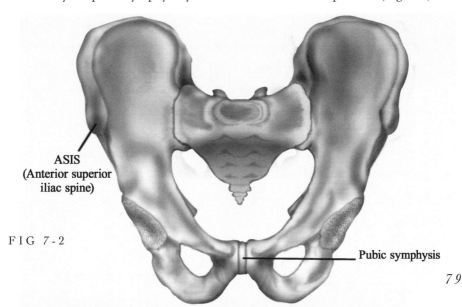

ASIS
(Anterior superior
iliac spine)

Pubic symphysis

FIG 7-2

79

You can check your position with a mirror (Fig. 7-3).

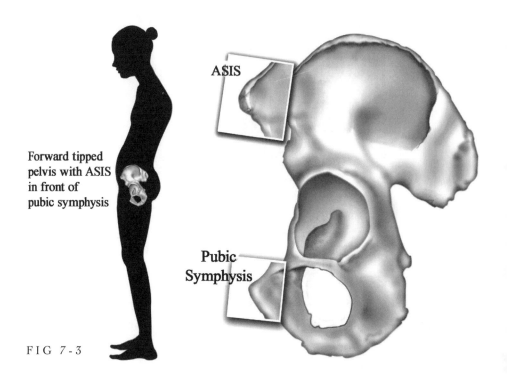

Forward tipped
pelvis with ASIS
in front of
pubic symphysis

ASIS

Pubic
Symphysis

FIG 7-3

TURN-OUT AND FEMORAL ANTEVERSION

Most dancers in classical ballet are concerned about how many degrees of turn-out they might have at the hip. Turn-out is what happens when you go from feet parallel in front of you to your toes pointing out away from you. Active turn-out occurs from the hip—in the hip socket.

There is a high degree of variation in the amount of turn-out that individual dancers can achieve. And although dancers and their teachers tend to obsess over the amount of turn-out available at the hip, 40–50% of your turn-out actually comes naturally without forcing your joints from your tibia and foot. However, your hip joint bony anatomy is important to determining how much natural turn-out you will be able to achieve.

It is helpful to think about your femur as a Popsicle stick and a ball earring with a pin (Fig. 7-4).

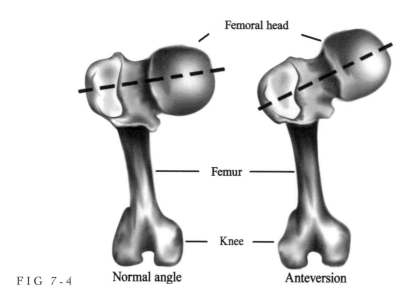

Femoral head

Femur

Knee

FIG 7-4   Normal angle   Anteversion

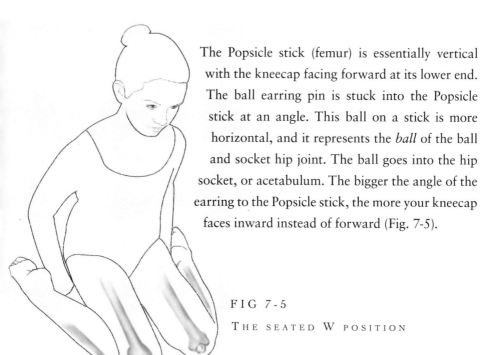

The Popsicle stick (femur) is essentially vertical with the kneecap facing forward at its lower end. The ball earring pin is stuck into the Popsicle stick at an angle. This ball on a stick is more horizontal, and it represents the *ball* of the ball and socket hip joint. The ball goes into the hip socket, or acetabulum. The bigger the angle of the earring to the Popsicle stick, the more your kneecap faces inward instead of forward (Fig. 7-5).

FIG 7-5

THE SEATED W POSITION

81

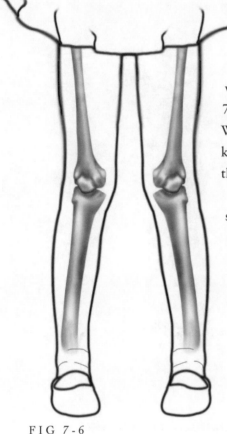

FIG 7-6

This is called *anteversion*. If you think about it, if the angle of the femoral head to your femur is high and you have increased anteversion, you will also have naturally less turn-out (Fig. 7-6; Magee 2002, 622–623, 625). The seated W position places considerable force on the knee and should be generally be avoided by the dancer.

It is just geometric reality. Is this a disaster? No. Does it mean you have to be more careful about stretches for your hip? Yes. It also means that you may be tempted to try to sway your low back to increase your turn-out or wing your feet. These are not good ideas!

Your turn-out does not just come from your hip. Turn-out can also happen at the hip, the knee, and even the foot! Not forcing the turn-out means you are not *using compensatory movements* from your foot, knee, or low back to increase the apparent scope of your turn-out. When you force the turn-out, you increase the risk of injuring yourself (Howse 2000, 187–192). Neuromuscular control and balance are the key to dancing without injury. If you are not forcing your turn-out, you will have a better overall dance look as well as more stability. Dancers who force the turn-out by winging their feet, swaying their low back, or torquing their knees sacrifice this control and increase the risk of long-term injury.

Hip Muscles

In the bowl of your pelvis, in front of the hip joint, is a large muscle called the *iliopsoas muscle*. The iliopsoas muscle flexes your thigh, for example, in front développé or battement—or even normal walking. There are other muscles that flex the hip but the iliopsoas is a common cause of groin pain in dancers. We will talk about that in greater detail later in the chapter.

Behind the hip, the gluteus maximus and hamstrings are powerful hip extensors. You use the gluteus maximus to assist with arabesque, for example. Also behind the hip is a group of short but strong muscles that rotate the hip (Fig. 7-7).

The piriformis, obturator internus, obturator externus, gemellus superior and inferior, and quadratus femoris muscles all externally rotate your hip and assist with your turn-out. The piriformis is another common cause of hip pain in dancers. More about that soon!

Inside the thigh are the adductors longus, brevis, and magnus. These all pull the femur to the midline. The pectineus and the gracilis assist these muscles. Strains of the inner thigh muscles are common and are one type of groin strain.

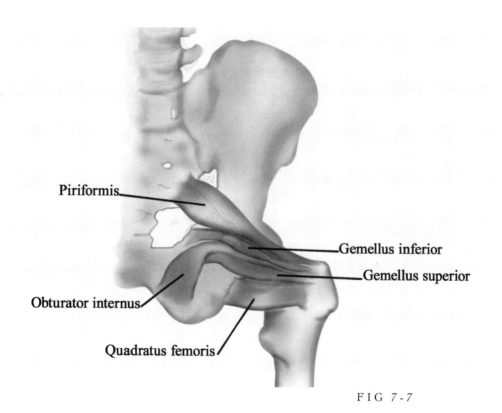

Piriformis

Gemellus inferior

Gemellus superior

Obturator internus

Quadratus femoris

FIG 7-7

Finally, the outside of the thigh has the gluteus medius and minimus. These muscles pull the thigh away from the midline. Also found on the outer hip is the muscle the *tensor fascia lata* with its tendon called the *iliotibial band* or *ITB band* (Fig. 7-8).

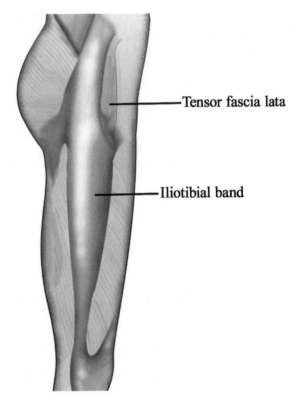

Tensor fascia lata

Iliotibial band

FIG 7-8

CLICKING HIPS: ANTERIOR, LATERAL, AND POSTERIOR CLICKING

My hip clicks in front

There is a ligament called the *inguinal ligament* that the iliopsoas has to pass under. In side or front développé, the tendon of the iliopsoas can get frayed and irritated by this tendon, resulting in iliopsoas tendonitis. If your hip is clicking or popping in the front, toward the groin, you might have this problem (Melamed and Hutchinson 2002, 171). Sometimes, this is called an *internal snapping hip* because it sits toward the inside of your thigh.

If you have hip snapping in front, a physical therapist can help with hip flexor stretches and ultrasound. Dancers who have a narrow pelvis may be at increased risk of developing this problem. Many times, dancers with a hip that snaps in front have a very tight iliopsoas muscle. If these dancers had proper treatment earlier, however, the clicking would never have developed!

Any dancer with hip pain in front, however, should be checked by a doctor. Hip pain in a dancer may be the first sign of a stress fracture of the femur or the hip—and would require the dancer to rest so the fracture does not cause become more pronounced and with potential long lasting health issues (Fredrickson et al. 2006, 309). Dancers use the hip bones enough that the bone can get what is called a *fatigue fracture* (Connors and Sanz, 2009). In other words, the bone is so stressed beyond its ability to heal that it breaks down.

Your hip muscles may be too tight and weak to provide adequate shock absorption to protect the hip bones. Your calcium or vitamin D levels may have made your bones generally weaker than they should be. Whatever the reason for the stress fracture, femoral stress fractures need a specialist's attention because they can cause permanent hip problems and might even require surgical treatment to stabilize the bone.

My hip clicks on the side

The iliotibial band runs from your lateral (side) hip to your knee. Underneath the iliotibial band is the hip ball and socket joint. If your iliotibial band, or ITB, is too tight, it will start to click and snap as it goes over the head of the femur. This is a lateral clicking hip. Your physical therapist can stretch your ITB and help resolve this issue.

Piriformis syndrome: My hip hurts in back— near or in my buttock

The deep rotator muscles get a workout in dance. Fifth position, second position, side passé, deep plié, jeté. Just about every movement that you can think of places stress on the deep, strong piriformis that sits behind your hip. Piriformis syndrome is a real pain in the buttock! You will have pain and tightness with all turn-out. In addition, your leg may feel numb or weak from pressure of the piriformis muscle on the sciatic nerve.

Stretching is a big help. A physical therapist needs to assess your pelvic rotation in dance while you are at the barre. Some people may even need injections near the muscle to quiet down the inflammation. Solving this problem permanently will frequently require dancers to be retrained in how to use the deep rotator muscles of the hip. Frequently, weakness and a lack of coordination in the foot and ankle or other thigh muscles lead to the muscle strain of the piriformis. All of the injections in the world will not be a permanent cure without correct assessment, restorative therapy, and reeducation.

INJURIES TO THE LIGAMENTS OF THE HIP:
Labral tears and femoroacetabular impingement

My hip just hurts! And it feels like it is locking!

The hip socket is ringed by cartilage called the *labrum*, which helps stabilize the hip joint by making the socket deeper. The labrum also helps with shock absorption at your hip. The femoral head can press up too tight into the labrum causing painful or range-of-motion-limiting femoroacetabular impingements. The labrum can then develop flaps and tears. Sometimes these flaps and tears cause groin pain or clicking and locking in the hip.

There is a great deal of interest in treating these tears with arthroscopic surgery. The theory is that the hip arthroscopy and cleaning of microtears of the cartilage that holds the femoral head in the joint will decrease the risk of arthritis in that joint in the future. There are really no long-term studies, however, to prove that this is the case. Very few studies have yet been published on dancers returning to dance after hip arthroscopic surgery. Although some of the initial data shows that some dancers may benefit from this type of surgery, there is very little long-term follow-up of dancer patients treated arthroscopically in the literature (Kocher et al. 2006, 102,103).

Dancers are not like other athletes! Your need for range of motion at your hip is very different, for example, from a football linebacker. So be very very cautious about the studies that are quoted to show that hip arthroscopy is successful in athletes. You care that this surgery works for YOU!

I would personally be very cautious about this type of surgical intervention at the present time. Prior to any such surgical intervention, please get a second and even a third surgical opinion. In addition, see a physical therapist and physician who specialize in dance medicine and have a broad range of experience in treating the hip.

MRI evaluation can be helpful in visualizing these tears. There are specific MRI scan sequences that give better detail of the labrum. If you have acute hip pain that radiates toward the groin, it is possible that you have acutely torn the labrum. Get yourself the best advice on how to heal an isolated labral tear.

The older dancer or the dance teacher with hip pain

Hip arthritis is common in dance teachers. The hip feels stiff; the teacher cannot close in fifth; the teacher cannot move as quickly across the dance space.

Hip X-rays do not tell the complete story in hip osteoarthritis. If you are stiff, if you have hip pain—and particularly groin pain—remember that cartilage does not image well on plain X-ray and that MRI with very specific sequences may be necessary to get you the information about arthritis that you need. Exercises to restore hip muscular balance help most older dancers with hip arthritis.

It is worth thinking about an anti-inflammatory diet, which includes fresh fruits and vegetables such as tomatoes, berries, and mushrooms. Fish such as salmon, high in omega-3 fatty acids, are also thought to be anti-inflammatory. Try to use extra-virgin olive oil instead of corn oil for cooking.

Glucosamine and chondroitin sulfate seem to help many people who suffer with arthritis pain. Acetaminophen and the anti-inflammatory medicines under a doctor's supervision can help, but they also can cause health problems, including potentially very severe liver injury. Although many of these medicines are over the counter—use them with caution and only as directed.

Dr. Vad of the Weill College of Cornell Medical University reports that 510 mg. of ginger with 1,500 mg. of glucosamine and 1,200 mg. of chondroitin gave helpful symptom control for his patients (Beaulé 2007, 17). Cortisone injections also are helpful for some patients.

Brief periods of use of a cane in the hand opposite to the painful hip can be helpful in severe flares. Aquatic exercise, which seems to be particularly beneficial for hip arthritis pain, is a generally good method to exercise while decreasing the stress on your knees, hips, and spine.

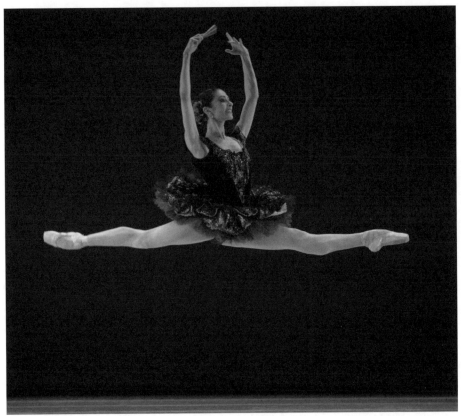

PENNSYLVANIA BALLET PRINCIPAL DANCER ARANTXA OCHOA IN MARIUS PETIPA'S
DON QUIXOTE. PHOTOGRAPH BY PAUL KOLNIK.

Five Important Facts about Your Hip

1. If you have a clicking hip, even if it is not painful, get it checked by a clinician.
   That clicking is a sign of tightness that may cause big problems down the road
   in your dance season or career.

2. Dancers who have been told they have femoroacetabular impingement or labral
   tears need to seek the advice of dance medicine professionals and do extensive
   supervised therapy prior to deciding on a surgical course of treatment for this
   problem. It is not yet clear what the long-term results of these surgeries will be
   for dancers because of the extreme demands dance puts on the hips.

3. Hip pain in front is often from iliopsoas tendonitis—and lunges can really
   be effective in loosening up the muscle. Iliopsoas tendonitis is often a sign
   of muscular imbalance at the hip. A dance physical therapist will be able to
   assess if you have forced the turn-out or are tipping your pelvis. Strengthening

and ultrasound will be of help. Be aware also that hip pain in front can be in the bones. You need to find out if there is a stress fracture in your hip before beginning a course of exercise and stretching for this type of pain.

4. Hip pain on the side can be from iliotibial tendonitis and better stretching and foam rollers can be a huge help. Ultrasound and myofascial release work are often tremendously effective. If your iliotibial band tendonitis stubbornly refuses to settle down, cortisone shots can be hugely successful in these selected cases in helping with pain.

5. Hip pain in the back can be piriformis syndrome. Hot tub soaks and stretching of the external rotators of the hip can alleviate the symptoms.

Five Really Awesome Hip Exercises and Stretches for Dancers

1. Lunges stretch the hip flexors and can even be done from a chair. Karen Clippinger describes a stretch in which the dancer has one knee on a chair with the stance leg in front. The dancer bends the stance leg to feel the stretch in the front of the other hip (Clippinger 2007, 224). Remember—if your hip flexors are too tight your pelvis will tip to the front. This is a great stretch to decrease your tendency toward a tipped pelvis and low back pain.

2. Hamstring stretches: sit in a chair with your legs extended in front of you about shoulders–width apart. Keep your knees slightly bent. Now bring your nose over one knee and count to 20. Roll up and then bring your nose down to the midline. Roll up and then bring your nose down over the other knee. Roll back up to neutral. Do this before and after dance.

3. The wall: lie on your back and rest your legs against a wall. Your legs should be in turned-out position. Your buttocks should be up against the wall. Slowly let your legs drop to the side and then slowly return them to the starting position of the V. You will feel a great stretch and also strengthen your thighs and hips.

4. Sit in a chair and cross your right leg so the ankle sits on your left knee. Press down with your hands on the right thigh near the knee to open up the hip and stretch. Now reverse.

5. The iliotibial band can become tight and cause hip, thigh, or knee pain. To stretch the right iliotibial band, stand so that you are perpendicular to a wall with your right hand on the wall. Your left hand will be on your left hip. Cross your left foot in front of and over your right foot. Bend your left knee and lean into your right hip. Lean your right hip into the wall while bending your left knee. The back, right leg will be straight. Hold 20-30 seconds. Repeat on the other side.

References

Beaulé, Paul E., MD, ed. 2007. "The Young Adult with Hip Pain." *American Academy of Orthopedic Surgeons, Monograph Series 38*, series edited by Peter Amadio, MD. Rosemont, IL: American Academy of Orthopaedic Surgeons.

Chow, Alex Hung Lit and William B. Morrison. 2011. "Imaging of Hip Injuries in Dancers." *Journal of Dance Medicine and Science* 15 (2, June).

Connors, John F. and Ana J. Sanz. 2009. "A Guide to Hip Injuries and Lower Extremity Ramifications in Female Athletes." *Podiatry Today* 22 (8, August). http://www.podiatrytoday.com/a-guide-to-hip-injuries-and-lower-extremity-ramifications-in-female-athletes.

Deckert, Jennifer L. "Improving Pelvic Alignment." 2009. *The IADMS Bulletin for Teachers* 1(1): 11-12.

Fredericson, Michael, MD, Fabio Jennings, MD, Christopher Beaulieu, MD, PhD. and Gordon O. Matheson, MD, PhD. 2006. "Stress Fractures in Athletes." *Topics in Magnetic Resonance Imaging* 17 (5, October): 309–325.

Heist, Lauren. "Don't Let Arthritis Keep You Out of the Classroom." *Dance Teacher.* http://www.dance-teacher.com/content/dont-let-arthritis-keep-you-out-classroom.

Howse, Justin. 2000. *Dance Technique and Injury Prevention,* third edition. New York: Routledge.

Kocher, Mininder S., Ruth Solomon, B. Minsuk Lee, Lyle J. Micheli, John Solomon, and Allston Stubs. 2006. "Arthroscopic Debridement of Hip Labral Tears in Dancers." *Journal of Dance Medicine and Science* 10 (3–4): 99–105.

Magee, David J. 2002. *Orthopedic Physical Assessment,* fourth edition. Philadelphia, PA: W. B. Saunders Company.

Martinez, Nina MD; Steven Mandel, MD; and Judith R. Peterson, MD. 2011. "Neurologic Causes of Hip Pain in Dancers." *Journal of Dance Medicine and Science* 15 (2, June).

Melamed, Hooman, MD and Mark R. Hutchinson, MD. 2002. "Soft Tissue Problems of the Hip in Athletes." *Sports Medicine and Arthroscopy Review* 10 (2, June): 168–175.

Nazarian, Levon N. 2011. "Musculoskeletal Ultrasound: Applications in the Hip. *Journal of Dance Medicine and Science* 15 (2, June).

8 The Knee

BONES OF THE KNEE

Your knee is the single largest joint in your body. Imagine your life with a stiff knee as a dancer! Your ability to smoothly bend and extend the knee joint is critical to performance in dance.

Your knee (Fig. 8-1) starts with the long bone of your thigh, called the *femur*, and ends at the smaller bones of your lower leg, called the *tibia* and the *fibula*. The kneecap is probably the part of the knee that most people are familiar with because it is so close to the surface of your skin and you can feel it gliding back and forth. Your kneecap, or *patella*, actually rests within an extension of the quadriceps muscle in the front of your thigh and is tied to the lower leg by the patellar ligament.

MUSCLES OF THE KNEE

Your knee predominately extends (straightens) and flexes (bends). Your lower leg also rotates but that is not the primary movement we think of at the knee. When

FIG 8-1

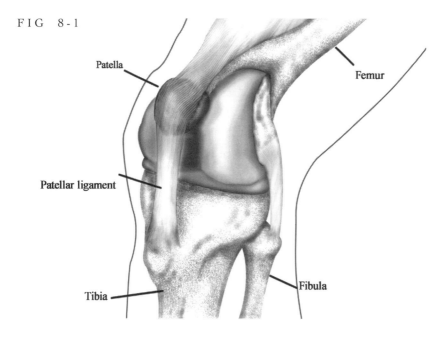

Patella

Femur

Patellar ligament

Tibia

Fibula

you straighten, or extend, your knee, the huge muscles in front of your thigh powerfully contract. This quadriceps muscle group is really four muscles that act together in the front of the knee (Fig. 8-2).

FIG 8-2

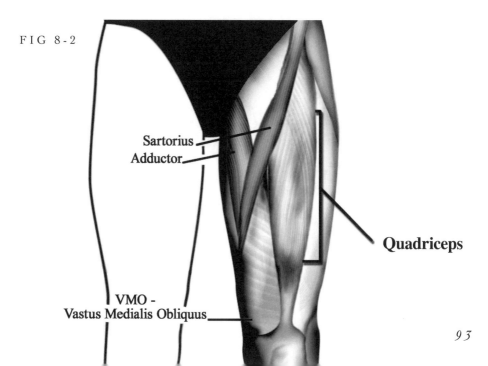

Sartorius
Adductor

Quadriceps

VMO -
Vastus Medialis Obliquus

The quadriceps muscle even helps control the knee as you bend, so you do not just collapse all at once into flexion (Trepman et al. 1998). This type of lengthening contraction is called an *eccentric contraction*. The large quadriceps also assists turn-out through the actions of the vastus medialis obliquus (VMO) which is on the inner thigh near the kneecap. This part of the quadriceps is a continuation of thigh muscles called the *adductors* that work at the hip to help your turn-out. In addition, the VMO helps keep your kneecap from sliding out of the groove in which it normally glides.

Muscles toward the inner knee

The *sartorius* muscle is a muscle from your hip that attaches to your knee below the joint line on the inside. Any movement of your thigh during turn-out stretches this muscle. Where the muscle inserts on the lower leg, there is a bursa, or sac, that the muscle glides over as your lower leg turns. This bursa can get inflamed causing pain below the joint line on the inside of your knee. This is called *pes anserine bursitis*. If your turn-out is tight and you force it, you can have this problem (Fig. 8-3).

FIG 8-3

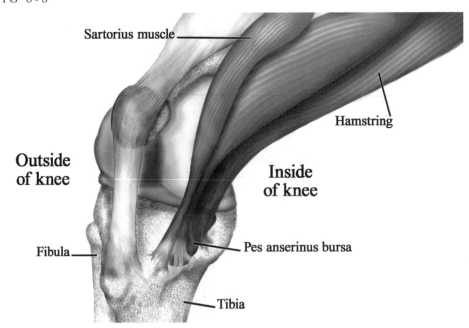

Sartorius muscle

Hamstring

Outside of knee

Inside of knee

Fibula

Pes anserinus bursa

Tibia

Muscles behind the knee

Behind the femur is the hamstring muscle group, which is very strong. These muscles flex, or bend, the knee. The outer part of the muscle attaches to the knee partly through the iliotibial band (ITB) that we talked about in Chapter 7 concerning the hip. When the hamstrings contract, your knee bends. If your hamstrings are too tight or not stretched well, you will have trouble with jetés. The hamstrings insert into your pelvis; so, when those muscles are tight, the pulling on your pelvis can affect your lumbar spine and low back, making them feel tight. If the back of your thighs are tight, you should stretch, stretch, stretch—and be sure to see your physical therapist if you do not get results (Clippinger 2007, 150).

FORCES ON THE KNEECAP

Your patella, or kneecap, is very important to how your knee functions. Your knee joint sits right between two of the longest bones in the body, the femur of your thigh and the tibia of your lower leg. Because the bones are long, the forces on the knee joint are fairly extreme. Your kneecap, or patella, allows your knee to be really strong when your leg is fully straight by allowing the big muscles in the front of your thigh to work more effectively while also spreading out the force of the contraction of those big muscles in the front of your thigh. This is a pretty neat trick! You get a stronger jump with less force on your knee joint when the patella is tracking straight and gliding smoothly.

PREDOMINANTLY ANTERIOR KNEE PAIN AND ITS CAUSES

Dancers' kneecaps: alignment issues of the leg and pain at the front of the knee

If you look carefully at the photos of the beautiful long legs of dancers, you begin to notice something peculiar. Many ballet dancers have knees that not only are fully extended when they stand, they are hyperextended (Fig. 8-4)!

Dr. Trepman and his colleagues studied how professional dancers' leg muscles work. Every single ballet dancer studied had this backward curve to the knee, a condition of the knee is called *genu recurvatum*, that translates to *knee backward bent*—a very accurate description of the condition. This condition

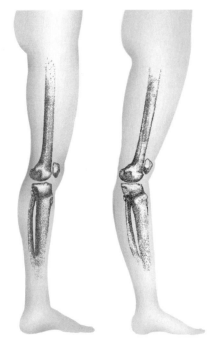

FIG 8-4

gives the leg a longer look than a single straight line from the hip to the foot might and it is certainly aesthetically delightful to look at. Some dancers also just lean back into their knees because it allows them to passively stand without pulling up through the leg. This enables the knee to lock without the dancer's exerting any effort—but it also gradually stretches out the back of the knee or posterior knee capsule.

Dancers with a knee that bows toward the back when they stand put a lot of force on the back of the kneecap, which can result in pain in the front of the knee. The forcing of the patella back against the femur, and the generally high number of dancers with genu recurvatum partly explains why front-of-the-knee pain is so common in dance. Karen Clippinger surveyed dancers and reported that almost 40% of professional or preprofessional dancers had been bothered by patellofemoral-type symptoms at the front of their knees (Clippinger 2007, 289).

Patellofemoral pain: Q who?

A recurved (recurvatum), or hyperextended, knee is not the only condition that can cause kneecap pain, or "patellofemoral pain syndrome." Another common kneecap issue that can contribute to this type of pain occurs if the kneecap, or patella, sits too far toward the outside of your leg. When this happens, the kneecap starts to bang against the edges of the groove that normally would help it to track and glide smoothly on your knee.

The Q angle (see Fig. 8-5) is the angle the long femur bone makes with the tendon that attaches your kneecap to the tibia. It is called the Q angle because the quadriceps muscle covers the femur. The Q angle is a factor that affects whether or not there is too much pressure on the outside of the kneecap. In reality, the Q angle is only one component of a very complicated story of the forces on the knee (Nguyen et al. 2009, 203). Some doctors do feel that a larger Q angle, which would imply a relatively wide pelvis, increases the force on the kneecap to move it to the outside and cause problems.

We are all born with a specific Q angle and there is not too much we can do to change that! But there are ways we can actively make our Q angle forces much worse. If you roll your foot to try to increase your turn-out, you will increase your Q angle, and this may increase the force on your kneecap (Fig. 8-5).

FIG 8-5

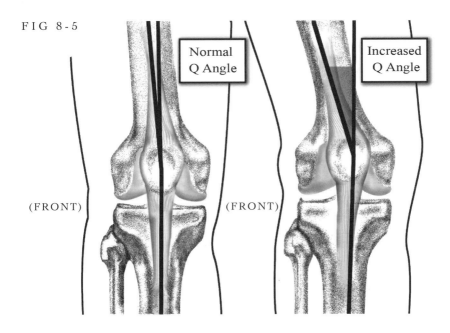

Normal Q Angle

Increased Q Angle

(FRONT)   (FRONT)

If you are a dancer who has problems with turn-out, forcing it in this way will not work out well for you. Instead, you will give yourself muscular imbalances, technique errors, and injury and pain. It is better to work with your teacher and physical therapist to get your turn-out working correctly.

Patellar dislocation

Because of the stress on the kneecap in dance, dance is high-risk activity for dislocating a kneecap. The kneecap basically can snap out of place. Typically, a young dancer in class starts or lands a jump and feels a pop in the knee; the knee is both painful and looks strange. Many times the kneecap will relocate to the correct placement without any doctor treating the knee. But the dancer will still be in quite a bit of pain in the front and at the sides of the kneecap. Any dancer whose kneecap has snapped out of place MUST see a doctor.

Why do dancers' kneecaps dislocate? There are many reasons a patella snaps out of place. Some dancers have a shallow groove for the patella to sit in so the kneecap can more easily slip out of its track. Some dancers have weaker inner thighs than they should, which allows the kneecap to be pulled too hard to the outside and jump out of its track. Some doctors think a higher Q angle increases the risk of patellar dislocation. Rolling your foot too much to flatten it to the floor will increase the stress on the kneecap and cause it to jump out of position. There are many reasons for a kneecap to move out of place!

It is not a good situation for a dancer when a patella has dislocated even if it goes back into place by itself—which is usually what happens. Sometimes when a kneecap has dislocated, part of the knee structure has fractured or broken —a condition that needs to be immediately assessed and treated. Also, if the dancer's knee is really swollen after the kneecap has moved out of place, there may be injury to the cartilage of the joint that would need to be evaluated by a doctor. And any kneecap that has dislocated once is very much at risk to repeat the behavior! So if your kneecap has dislocated you need to get a doctor to check your knee (Mehta et al. 2007, 78).

The good news is that most dancers who dislocate a patella for the first time will most likely not need surgery to tack the kneecap back into place. However, those dancers more than likely will need to immobilize their knee in a long leg splint and then get therapy to strengthen it. If a dancer does not get correct medical treatment for a kneecap dislocation, the patella could dislocate over and over again from chronic instability. As explained earlier, even without thinking about the kind of pain this would cause, each dislocation exposes the knee to the risk of developing permanent cartilage injury or a fracture. So treat your kneecap dislocation correctly by getting it checked (Fithian 2004, 1114).

PROBLEMS WITH THE LIGAMENTS AND MENISCI

The ligaments of your knee help keep the bones from sliding out of place when you jump, run, and walk. They keep your knee stable so you do not collapse on jumps or other movements (Fig. 8-6).

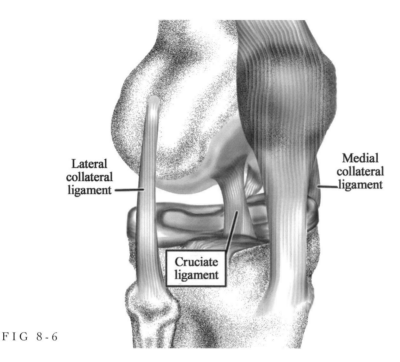

Lateral
collateral
ligament —

Medial
collateral
ligament

Cruciate
ligament

FIG 8-6

You can think of the ligaments as slightly stretchy ropes that tether the long bone, or femur, above the knee to the tibia and fibula below your knee. These ropes prevent the tibia and fibula of your lower leg from sliding too far forward or too far backward, or from collapsing inward or outward with too great an angle compared to your thigh. These are the four directions in which the lower leg could move too far away from the upper leg. So, not surprisingly, there are four important ligaments in the knee that prevent that from happening!

An important one for dancers to know about is the medial collateral ligament, which goes from your thigh to your lower leg on the inside of your knee. It prevents your knee from collapsing in when you stand. If you roll your foot in when you plié, you put stress on the inside of your knee and this ligament. During a plié at the barre, take a moment to see where your knee falls with respect to your foot. Your teacher has probably told you "keep that knee over that foot!" If a straight line down from your knee to the floor is closer to the midline of your body than the midline of your foot, you are stretching, straining, and stressing the inner knee, including the medial collateral ligament. Dancers who chronically stress the inner knee in this way at best end up with a less stable knee, increasing their risk of other knee injuries. Technique matters! Watch that foot and knee placement so you do not get a loose knee structure.

The lateral collateral ligament prevents the knee from bowing to the outside. The anterior and posterior cruciate ligaments prevent the lower leg from sliding too much forward or backward compared to the thigh. These ligaments are less often injured in dancers, however, than the medial collateral ligament (Fig. 8-7).

FIG 8-7

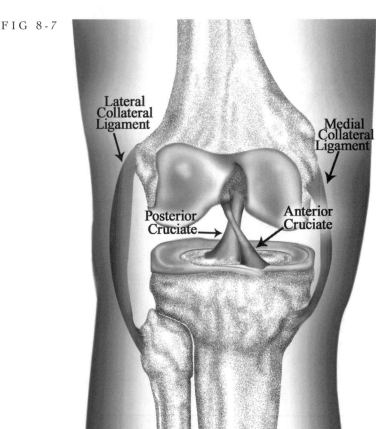

There are two menisci on the inside of your knee. The menisci are shock absorbers in between your thigh and lower leg bones (Fig. 8-8). The least you need to know about these complex structures is that the medial meniscus and lateral meniscus of your knee are pieces of cartilage that allow the knee to absorb the shocks of landings and pliés. These pieces of cartilage help the knee glide smoothly as you flex and bend your knee. Any injury or tear of these structures puts you at risk for additional short term and long term knee damage and pain (Bhagia, Weinik, and Xing 2009).

FIG 8-8

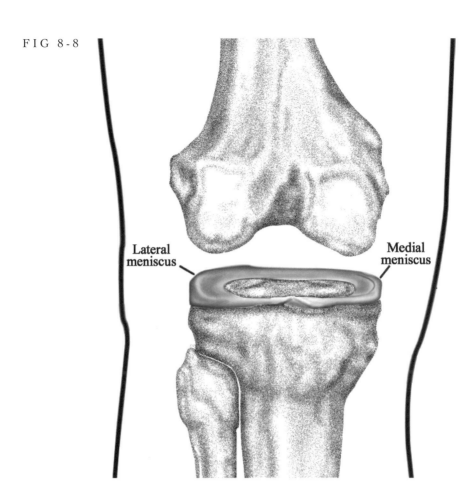

Lateral
meniscus

Medial
meniscus

The meniscus to the inside of your knee is called the *medial meniscus*. The meniscus to the outside of your knee is called the *lateral meniscus*. The medial meniscus is tacked down inside your knee while the lateral meniscus has a greater ability to glide.

Some doctors think it is the larger size along with the decreased mobility of the medial meniscus that puts it at so much risk. In addition, only its very outer rim gets a good blood supply, so you see why dancers are setups to injure the medial meniscus! Faulty jump landings put too much pressure on the inside of your knee. As a result, you could injure the medial meniscus as well as the medial collateral ligament. Jumps, pliés, turns—anything that stresses your knee stresses the medial meniscus.

If you injure your medial meniscus, you might feel pain along the joint line. Your joint might lock or you might feel as if you have to push to bend your knee. Your knee may swell. A piece of the meniscus may even block smooth movement of your joint to the extent that you feel like your joint is locking or popping.

If you think you have a meniscus injury, it is good to get it checked by a doctor. Proper rehab can do wonders for injury to your meniscus. Blood supply to the meniscus is relatively poor and healing from this type of injury can take well over a month—even if you do not need surgery to repair it. Whether or not to have surgery to repair a torn meniscus is a very individual decision based on your ability to dance (and do everything else you and your knee want to do), your pain, and the type of meniscal tear you have.

If you suspect you tore a meniscus or injured your meniscus, get treatment to help prevent further tears or injury.

ANOTHER STRUCTURE: THE PLICA

Some dancers and athletes are told they have a meniscal injury, get treated, but still have problems. Some dancers even get surgery to repair a meniscus and yet that nagging pain on the inside of their knee persists.

Separate from the ligaments and the meniscus, there is yet another structure on the inside of dancers' knees that frequently causes pain. This structure is called the *plica*, developmental embryonic soft tissue (that usually goes away) on the inner knee at the joint line. Approximately 10% of adults have the plica as a remnant that persists inside the joint (Rue, Ferry, and Bach 2008).

The plica can become irritated and scarred and can cause the knee to have painful impingement. If you feel local tenderness to the inside of your patellar ligament, you might actually have an inflamed plica. Hamstring stretches and treatment with anti-inflammatory medication such as ibuprofen are very helpful for inflammation of the plica. Your doctor may inject anesthetics and steroids to settle down plica irritation while you do rehab. It is important to remember that not all inner knee pain is from a ligament sprain or meniscal tear, so remember to always get this type of pain checked by your doctor.

PAIN AT THE OUTSIDE OF THE KNEE

We have talked about pain at the front of the knee and pain at the sides of the knees. The most common reason dancers get pain on the outside of the knee is from the iliotibial band getting into trouble from friction (Fig. 8-9).

FIG 8-9

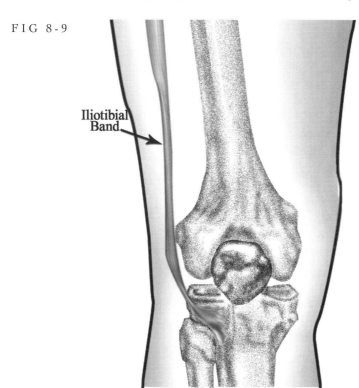

Iliotibial
Band

Quadriceps and patellar tendonitis

The quadriceps muscle is really a group of four muscles in the front of your thigh that powerfully straightens your knee and allows you to jump high and really control your landings well. The quadriceps tendon connects to your kneecap, or patella, and then continues below the patella to the tibial tubercle (Fig. 8-10).

As you can imagine, these muscles and tendons get overworked by dancers. If you have suddenly increased your time spent dancing, you can overstress these structures and develop pain.

Jumper's knee is another term for *patellar tendonitis*. Tendonitis is a painful inflammation of the tissue that attaches a muscle to a bone. Do I need to tell you

FIG 8-10

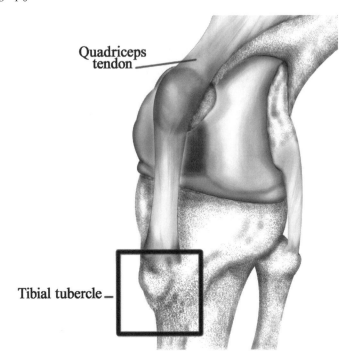

Quadriceps
tendon

Tibial tubercle

which dance movements put you at risk for the painful syndrome below your
knee? Yes, jumping will put you at risk for jumper's knee! Hamstring stretches
and quadriceps stretches help to avoid strains of the patellar tendon. A tight calf
muscle means you have to load your quadriceps muscles even more to attain height
in jumps, so stretching the calf muscle helps as well.

KNEE ARTHROSCOPY

If you have knee instability, if your knee locks or pops, or if you have ongoing pain
in your knee despite physical therapy, you may need to have a surgeon surgically
put probes into your knee to directly visualize the structures and, hopefully, get
any anatomical problems corrected. Surgery is a big step and, for the vast majority
of knee injuries related to dance, is not necessary; most dancers' knee issues can
be adequately visualized with plain X-ray and with MRI. MRI gives incredibly
detailed images of the entire knee joint, so most of the time your doctors will be
able to give you a treatment plan by using this type of imaging technique.

KNEE ARTHRITIS

Arthritis of the knee can occur after a trauma, such as a hard fall on your knee, or from wear and tear after years of dance. The joint surfaces become irregular and grind together causing pain. The menisci that we discussed earlier literally break down with tears and fissures. The ligaments become frayed and stretched.

Keeping the muscles of your joint strong will help to prolong the life of that joint. If you have chronic pain from arthritis, acetaminophen and other anti-inflammatory medicine such as ibuprofen can help with symptom control. Although the use of over-the-counter medicines like glucosamine and chondroitin sulfates is controversial, many patients experience significant relief of pain from them and some medical studies support their use. Credible evidence demonstrates that acupuncture done by qualified providers helps alleviate knee pain from osteoarthritis.

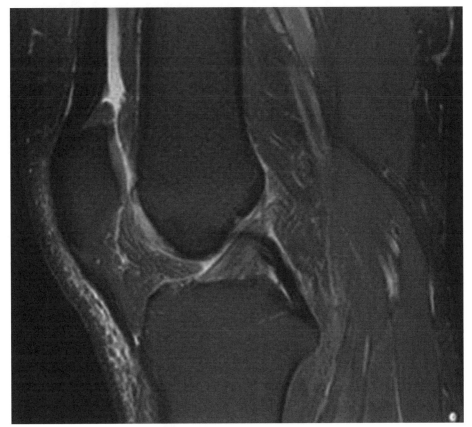

MRI, NORMAL SAGITTAL IMAGE OF KNEE. COURTESY THOMAS JEFFERSON UNIVERSITY HOSPITAL, PHILADELPHIA, PA.

If your joint cracks, creaks, and is painful with every step, you may want to discuss *viscosupplementation* or a cortisone shot in your knee with your doctor. Viscosupplementation is a long medical term for "placing artificial joint fluid back into your knee with a syringe." This is done in an outpatient setting and can help restore the bounce to your knee joint. The artificial joint fluid provides the knee with better shock absorption and therefore reduces knee pain caused by moving the knee.

Finally, exercising in water decreases stress on the joint and may be very helpful. Aquatic rehabilitation, or water exercise, works because you are able to exercise without loading the joint as extensively. We are buoyant in water, and so you will be able to exercise fairly well without a great deal of joint stress.

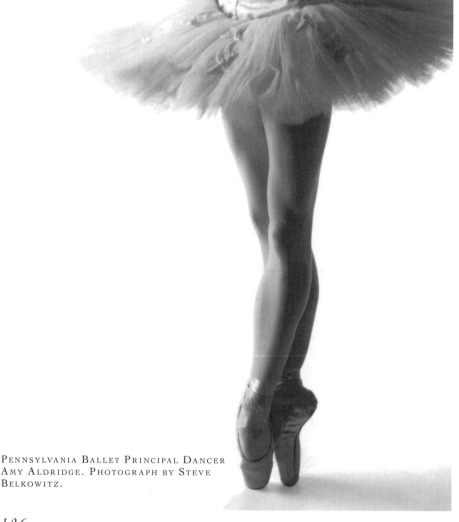

PENNSYLVANIA BALLET PRINCIPAL DANCER
AMY ALDRIDGE. PHOTOGRAPH BY STEVE
BELKOWITZ.

Five Critical Things to Know about Your Knee

1. The knee is enormously complicated. If you are having pain or stiffness, locking, or popping, get it checked. Your knee health is fundamental to your health as a dancer.

2. Most pain in the front of the knee is from patellofemoral syndrome. Many people with patellofemoral syndrome can be helped with correct stretching and muscle strength rebalancing.

3. Pain on the inside of the knee at the joint line in dancers may be a medial collateral ligament strain. If you are forcing your turn-out, you may be stressing this ligament and giving yourself problems.

4. Most pain immediately below the knee is patellar tendonitis. Dancers who have suddenly increased the number of jetés they do, and dancers who work on floors that are too soft—floors without enough bounce and spring— can develop this problem. Make sure you stretch your quadriceps muscle. For the short term, consider a patellar ligament brace if your knee is very painful.

5. Tight hamstrings are a real problem for dancers. Tight hamstrings make it harder to do big jumps, increase the forces on the knee, and can cause some dancers to develop low back issues.

Five Great Knee Exercises

1. Wall slides: standing, place your back against the wall and your feet about one foot away from it. Your feet should be shoulder width apart. Slide up and down the wall without locking your knees. Do 20 repetitions, 2–3 times a day.

2. Squats: squat and press up. Do 20 repetitions, 3 times a day. Avoid knee flexion past 90 degrees (remember, bending your knee too deeply causes stress on the back of your kneecap). This can be done with or without a light bar weight across the shoulders. Your feet should be a comfortable distance apart and not extremely turned out. A personal trainer can help with your alignment for this exercise.

3. Walking lunges around a track: start slowly with this exercise, because your thighs will tire quickly when you first start. A reasonable beginning is 1 to 3 sets of approximately 10 lunges, then build up your endurance slowly. Turn around and return to where you started.

4. Lateral step-ups: stand on a comfortably wide platform, approximately one foot high. Start by standing with your weight on the right foot and touch down to the floor softly with your left foot. Then bring the left foot back up to the platform and either tap the left foot or pause for a second to stand if that helps you get your center. Then repeat by gently touching the left foot down to the floor again. Lower and raise your body smoothly. Do 20 step-ups this way. Switch legs and repeat.

5. Hamstring stretches: these are done sitting in chair with your legs straightened out in front of you in a V. Keep your knees slightly bent and lean forward over the right leg. Relax back to neutral. Repeat, bending down the middle. Repeat again, stretching forward over the left leg.

References

Bencardino, Jenny T., Zehava S. Rosenberg, Robert R. Brown, Alvand Hassankhani, Elizabeth S. Lustrin, and Javier Beltran. 2000. "Traumatic Musculotendinous Injuries of the Knee: Diagnosis with MR Imaging." *RadioGraphics* 20: S103–S120.

Bhagia, Sarjoo M., MD, Michael Weinik, DO, and Selina Yingqi Xing, MD, MS. 2009. "Meniscal Injury." *eMedicine from WebMD.com,* updated June 30. http://emedicine.medscape.com/article/308054-print.

Clippinger, Karen Sue. 2007. *Dance Anatomy and Kinesiology.* Champaign, IL: Human Kinetics.

Fithian, Donald C., Elizabeth W. Paxton, Mary Lou Stone, Patricia Silva, Daniel K. Davis, David A. Elias, and Lawrence M. White. 2004. "Epidemiology and Natural History of Acute Patellar Dislocation." *The American Journal of Sports Medicine* 32 (5, July): 1114–1121.

Gerbino, Peter F., Elizabeth D. Griffin, Pierre A. d'Hemecourt, Thomas Kim, Mininder Kocher, David Zurakowski, and Lyle J. Micheli. 2006. "Patellofemoral Pain Syndrome: Evaluation of Location and Intensity of Pain." *The Clinical Journal of Pain* 22 (2, February): 154–159.

Khan, Karim, Janet Brown, Sarah Way, Nicole Vass, Ken Crichton, Ron Alexander, Andrew Baxter, Marie Butler, and John Wark. 1995. "Overuse Injuries in Classical Ballet—Review." *Sports Medicine* 19 (5 May): 341–357.

Mehta, Vishal, Motoyasu Inoue, Eiki Nomura, and Donald C. Fithian. 2007. "An Algorithm Guiding the Evaluation and Treatment of Acute Primary Patellar Dislocations." *Sports Medicine and Arthroscopy Review* 15 (2, June): 78–81.

Nguyen, Anh-Dung, PhD, ATC; Michelle C. Boling, PhD, ATC; Beverly Levine, PhD; and Sandra J. Shultz, PhD, ATC. 2009. "Relationships Between Lower Extremity Alignment and the Quadriceps Angle." *Clinical Journal of Sport Medicine* 19 (3, May): 201–206.

Rue, John-Paul H., MD; Amon T. Ferry, MD; and Bernard R. Bach, Jr., MD. 2008. "Plica Excision, Revisited." *Techniques in Knee Surgery* 7 (1, March): 48–50.

Trepman, Elly, Richard E. Gellman, Lyle J. Micheli, and Carlo De Luca. 1998. "Electromyographic Analysis of Grand-Plié in Ballet and Modern Dancers." *Medicine and Science in Sports and Exercise* 30 (12, December): 1708–1720.

9 The Ankle and Socket Joint

E VERYONE KNOWS WHERE THE ANKLES ARE, RIGHT? THOSE BIG BONES THAT STICK OUT ON THE INNER AND OUTER LOWER LEG IS YOUR ANKLE. WELL, YES AND NO.

THE ANKLE JOINT IS REALLY MORE THAN ONE JOINT. THERE ARE TWO MOTIONS IN THE ANKLE THAT ARE IMPORTANT FOR DANCE AND THEY HAPPEN IN DIFFERENT PLACES.

THE MORTISE OF THE ANKLE JOINT

The ankle joint proper, or the upper ankle joint, consists of the tibia (inner bump), the talus, and the fibula (outer bump). This part of the ankle joint is called the *ankle mortise* (Fig. 9-1). Most of the movement at this upper part of the joint is up and down—the motions that allow plié and pointe.

FIG 9-1

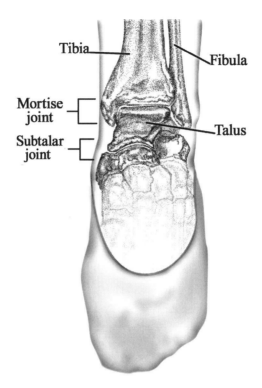

THE SUBTALAR JOINT

You can do this interesting experiment on your leg: Put a colored dot on the front of your leg. Now go onto full pointe—in other words stretch that foot toward the floor. The dot is not facing forward anymore, is it? It is facing more toward the outside now. That is because of the lower section of the ankle that sits below the ankle mortise. The bottom of the talus is called the *subtalar joint*. The ankle motion at this joint is to mostly roll the foot to the inside or outside.

This rotating motion of the leg allows the foot to pronate and supinate. When the foot is pronated, it is floppy and gets quite flat on the floor. A floppy, flat foot is a good shock absorber. When your foot is supinated, your arch is lifted off the floor and your foot becomes quite rigid. When you are on pointe, for example, you do not want a floppy foot; you want a rigid foot to keep you nice and upright. If you point your foot toward the floor to prepare to go on pointe or demi-pointe, your leg bone naturally rotates to the outside and your foot supinates slightly and therefore becomes more rigid. Nice how that works out, isn't it? Your body just wants you to dance.

ANKLE MOBILITY REQUIRED FOR DANCE

If you were a regular person—not a dancer—normal range of motion for your ankle is about 40–55 degrees of motion flexing the foot down, or plantarflexing, and about 10–20 degrees of motion bending the foot up, or dorsiflexing. But that amount of flexibility is not going to work well for dance. To get your foot to pointe nicely, your ankle needs to plantarflex 90–100 degrees—approximately double what a normal ankle range of motion is thought to be.

Osteoarthritis

Because the ankle is under so much stress in dance, ankle injuries happen fairly often. Researchers did an MRI study of Royal Ballet of Canada dancers who had danced professionally for approximately eight years and found arthritic change in dancers who were entirely asymptomatic (Salonen et al., 1999). None of the participants in this study were experiencing any ankle problems or pain, yet evidence of osteoarthritis existed in many of the dancers.

THE LIGAMENTS OF THE ANKLE

Ligaments help bones stay nicely in place by tying bones together like ropes. The ligaments to the outside are the ones most often stretched or sprained (Fig. 9-2).

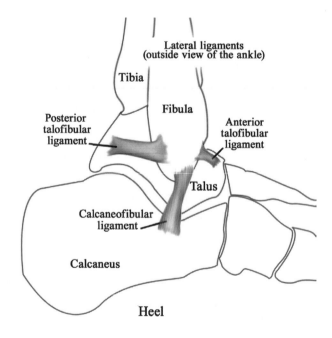

FIG 9-2

If you go up on pointe, fall off your pointe, and then have pain and swelling on the outside of your ankle, it is usually because you have sprained the lateral ligaments of your ankle. A sprained ankle means that one or more of the ligaments that support the ankle have been stretched or torn.

There are some simple rules you should follow if you have an ankle sprain. Immediately apply ice, and then rest. Next, apply compression with an elastic bandage or ace wrap and keep the ankle elevated. Remember not to apply ice directly to your skin; use a towel underneath the ice pack. This treatment is often referred to as RICE—rest, ice, compression, elevation.

If you cannot walk on the ankle immediately, or if you heard or felt a pop or snap in your ankle, you need to see a doctor as soon as possible. You could have fractured a bone.

Proprioception is our sense of where we are in space. It is very important for dancers to have balance rehabilitation or *proprioceptive* rehabilitation as well as regaining strength. If you fall off the ankle that was sprained more frequently or easily than you fall off the ankle that was not injured, you need additional rehabilitation exercise to restore your sense of balance. As part of their rehabilitation of lateral ankle sprains, dome dancers do single leg balance exercises on foam rubber soft mats in order to challenge their balance.

You need to work on balance exercises after you have an ankle sprain, even if your ankle is pain free (Small 2009, 317; Hudson 2009, 204). Try balancing on one foot and then on one foot with your eyes closed, using a barre or other supporting surface to balance if you fall off (Omey and Micheli, 1999).

After rehab of even a minor sprain, do not just rely on a doctor or physical therapist to check your strength or your ankle mobility and to tell you to return to dance. Dancers who do not get adequate rehab of ankle sprains become dancers who sprain their ankles again and again (Ferran, Oliva, and Maffulli 2009, 141). Do not let this be you!

The ligaments on the outside of the foot are the ones most commonly injured in an ankle sprain. But those are not the only important ligaments of your ankle. There is a ligament on the inside of your ankle that is important. This is called the *deltoid ligament.*

If your foot is forced out away from your body and then you have pain on the inside of your ankle, you might have sprained this deltoid ligament. Deltoid

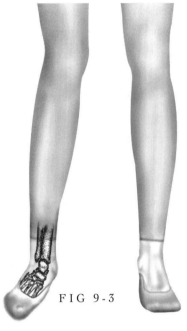

FIG 9-3

ligament sprains in dance should be fairly uncommon unless you have a pretty major fall that rotates your foot to the outside or are a chronic hyperpronator who rolls the foot too much to the inside. Dancers who roll the foot chronically are often subconsciously trying to force the turn-out. Your dance teacher and physical therapist will know if you are forcing your turn-out by rolling your foot too much (Fig. 9-3).

In the lower part of your ankle, the subtalar joint that allows you to roll your foot in or out (pronate and supinate) has another ligament that is very important to dancers. This ligament is called the *spring ligament* (Fig. 9-4; Clippinger 2007, 304).

The *plantar calcaneonavicular ligament* as it is called by its closest friends and foot and ankle surgeons, is a strap of ligament that goes from the navicular bone to the heel bone, or calcaneus. This ligament helps keep the arch elevated when you are standing. If you stretch this ligament too much, your foot is flatter

FIG 9-4

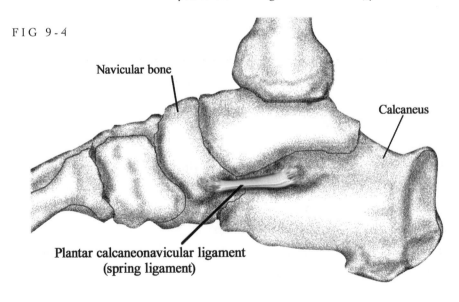

Navicular bone

Calcaneus

Plantar calcaneonavicular ligament
(spring ligament)

and floppier, making it more difficult for you to be stable on pointe. And if you have a very bad fall or misstep that forces your foot away from your body, you can tear this ligament, have your arch fall, and get severe pain toward the inside of your foot. If you have injured either the deltoid or the spring ligaments (Fig. 9-5), a doctor needs to help advise you on how best to rehabilitate and manage those injuries.

FIG 9-5

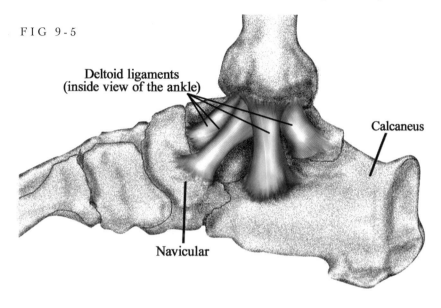

Deltoid ligaments
(inside view of the ankle)

Calcaneus

Navicular

Osteochondritis Dissecans: Diagnosis and Treatment

FIG 9-6

We talked about ankle sprains and their rehabilitation. If you have an ankle sprain that never seems to get better, even if the initial X-ray of your ankle was negative for any type of bone break, be sure to go back and speak with your doctor. Sometimes from trauma such as sprain, a tiny bone chip can break off the talus bone (Fig. 9-6).

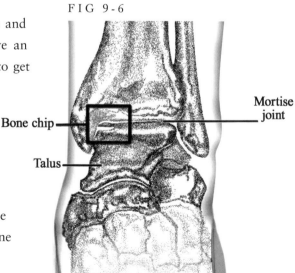

Bone chip

Talus

Mortise joint

When a dancer has a severe sprain, the talus can be forced up into the mortise of the joint, become severely bruised, and it sometimes even chips. This tiny chip and/or bruise sometimes does not show up on the initial X-ray. When this talus bone injury happens, sometimes the bone chip can heal back together with the rest of the bone if treated correctly. But if you ignore a bone chip, it can lose its blood supply. The bone chip then can never heal and it floats in your ankle joint causing grinding, popping, swelling and additional damage. This condition of a bone chip of the talus is called *osteochondritis dissecans*, which translates to "dry bone chip." The chip might need to be surgically treated or even removed from your joint. So if you feel a catching sensation in your ankle when you move your foot, or if you have persistent ankle pain after a sprain, even if your X-rays were negative, be sure to talk with your doctor about checking further for the problem of osteochondritis dissecans (Bowman 2008, 317–322).

BONY INJURY OF THE ANKLE AND ITS REHAB

Anterior ankle spurs

Deep ankle bends such as in grand pliés force the tibia bone against the talus. Over time, a dancer can develop bone spurs on the front of the ankle (Fig. 9-7).

These spurs can significantly decrease the dancer's ability to sink into grand plié and sometimes have to be surgically removed (Kennedy et al. 2008).

Posterior impingement and the os trigonum

As we discussed in the preceding section, some dancers have a buildup of soft tissue at the back of the ankle, making it hard for the dancer to go onto full pointe. As a result, the dancer "forces" the pointe (Hillier, Hulme, and Healy 2004, 532). Sometimes there is even a tiny piece of bone at the back of the ankle that blocks the dancer from getting to full pointe because of the posterior impingement. The bony block at the back of the ankle is a tiny particle of bone called the *os trigonum*. It can be found on X-rays even in dancers who do not have symptoms but it can really cause problems for some dancers' mobility in the ankle.

If you are having trouble getting onto full pointe, have a dance doctor see you and work with a physical therapist to improve your ankle flexibility. Anti-

FIG 9-7

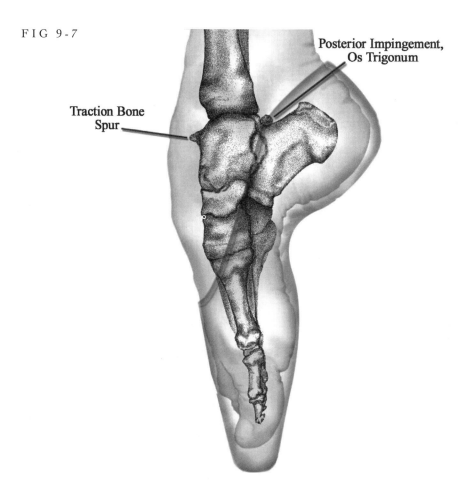

Posterior Impingement,
Os Trigonum

Traction Bone
Spur

inflammatory medicine is a temporary fix at best for this problem of os trigonum syndrome. Exercise that strengthens the other muscles besides the gastroc-soleus muscle (discussed in Chapter 11) that pull the foot onto pointe can be helpful. Ultrasound treatment can be very beneficial as well. You can discuss this with your physical therapist and dance medicine expert (Clippinger 2007, 368–369).

Anterior impingement

Ideally, to go into a really good and deep plié, dancers should have better than normal range for dorsiflexion (bringing your foot up) than most people. However, some studies seem to show that dancers do not have as good dorsiflexion range as they might want. Despite training, it is difficult for young ballet dancers to improve ankle dorsiflexion (Khan et al. 2000, 101).

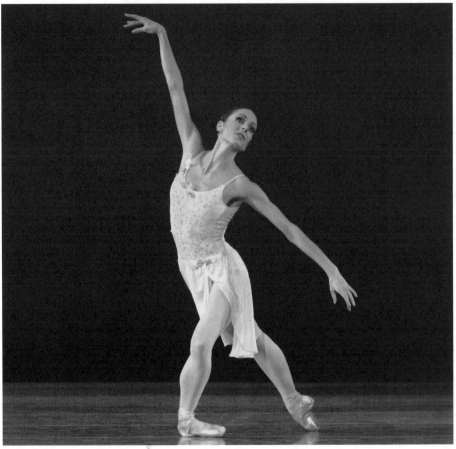

PENNSYLVANIA BALLET PRINCIPAL DANCER AMY ALDRIDGE IN GEORGE BALANCHINE'S *BALLO DELLA REGINA*. PHOTOGRAPGH BY PAUL KOLNIK.

Dancers who do not control their plié well and dancers who force their plié may develop chronic pain at the front of the ankle. Forcing the plié causes the tibia to shove into the talus bone over and over again. Done repeatedly, this can create a divot in the talus bone that sits in the ankle joint. The action creates soft tissue swelling at the front of the ankle and then the dancer needs to force the plié even more. This creates a terrible spiral of shallower and shallower pliés that require more force and cause more injury.

You can help stop this terrible cycle by not forcing your plié and by doing really good calf stretches—first with your knee straight and then with your knee bent. This makes sense because stretching those calf muscles will allow your ankle to dorsiflex with much less force, creating a deeper plié.

Five Critical Things to Know about Your Ankle

1. Your ankle moves up and down through the mortise and rolls side to side through the subtalar joint. The movement up is dorsiflexion and the movement down is plantarflexion. Dorsiflexion is important for plié and plantarflexion is important for pointe. Rolling in is pronation and rolling out is supination.

2. Pain at the outside of your ankle after a fall off pointe or an ankle twist is likely a sprain. If you cannot bear weight immediately after a sprain or the pain is severe, see a doctor. You may have a fracture.

3. Ankle sprains should generally be treated initially with RICE, which stands for Rest, Ice, Compression with an elastic bandage or ace wrap, and keeping the leg Elevated. Dance teachers may want to keep one pair of height adjustable crutches at the studio to help their students in the case of a sprain or leg injury.

4. An ankle sprain affects your balance. You need to rehab your balance even if you are pain free and move your ankle well. If you go back to dance when your balance is not fully recovered, you may sprain the ankle again and develop chronic instability. This unfortunate situation happens more frequently than you might think.

5. Pain that persists after an ankle sprain can be secondary to a bone chip—even if initial X-rays are negative. Make sure you see a doctor to get persistent ankle pain evaluated.

Six Great Exercises to Keep Your Ankles Strong and Flexible

1. Draw the alphabet with one foot while you are seated with the other foot planted on the ground. Repeat with the other foot.

2. While seated, get both feet up in the air and draw the alphabet with both feet simultaneously. Keep your feet moving together as symmetrically as possible to force your brain and feet to work together.

3. While you are standing at a supporting surface for balance if you need it, lift one foot off the ground. Stay as still as you can at the foot and ankle on the support side. Repeat with the other foot. Your goal is to see how long you can maintain your balance. Touch your hands down to regain balance when you feel yourself wobble.

4. Once exercise number three above gets easier, repeat it with your eyes closed.

5. Standing on one leg, slightly bend your supporting knee and then straighten it without locking it. See how many repetitions you can do without wobbling. Repeat with the other leg.

6. Dancers who are really strong can use a nonskid sock or sneaker and get up and down from the seated position on a high chair using one leg for support. Make sure that your chair cannot slide. Try not to collapse your knee to the inside or the outside. See how smoothly you can coordinate your thigh, leg, and ankle to get up and down from the chair softly without collapsing onto it.

References

Bowman, Michael. 2008. "Osteochondral Lesions of the Talus and Occult Fractures of the Foot and Ankle." In *Baxter's the Foot and Ankle in Sport*, second edition, edited by David A. Porter and Lew C. Schon, 317–322. Philadelphia, PA: Mosby, Inc.

Clippinger, Karen Sue. 2007. *Dance Anatomy and Kinesiology*. Champaign, IL: Human Kinetics.

Elias, Ilan, Adam C. Zoga, Steven M. Raikin, Judith R. Peterson, Marcus P. Besser, William B. Morrison, and Mark E. Schweitzer. 2008. "Bone Stress Injury of the Ankle in Professional Ballet Dancers Seen on MRI." *BMC Musculoskeletal Disorders* (March 28). http://www.biomedcentral.com.

Ferran, Nicholas A., MBBS, MRCS Ed; Francesco Oliva, MD, PhD, and Nicola Maffulli, PhD, FRCS. 2009. "Ankle Instability." *Sports Medicine and Arthroscopy Review* 17 (2, June): 139–145.

Hamilton, William G., Mihir M. Patel, and Roman A. Sibel. 2008. "Impingement Syndromes of the Foot and Ankle." In *Baxter's The Foot and Ankle in Sport,* second edition, edited by David A. Porter and Lew C. Schon, 29–44. Philadelphia, PA: Mosby, Inc.

Hiller, J. C., K. Peace, A. Hulme, and J. C. Healy. 2004. "MRI Features of Foot and Ankle Injuries in Ballet Dancers." *British Journal of Radiology* 77 (918, June): 532–537.

Hudson, Zoe, PhD. 2009. "Rehabilitation and Return to Play After Foot and Ankle Injuries in Athletes." *Medicine and Arthroscopy Review* 17 (3, September): 203–207.

Khan, Karim M., Kim Bennell, Selena Ng, Bernadette Matthews, Peter Roberts, Caroline Nattrass, Sarah Way, Janet Brown. April 2000. "Can 16–18-Year-Old Elite Ballet Dancers Improve Their Hip and Ankle Range of Motion Over a 12-Month Period?" *Clinical Journal of Sport Medicine,* 10:98–103.

Kennedy, John G., Christopher W. Hodgkins, Jean-Alain Columbier, and William G. Hamilton. 2008. "Foot and Ankle Injuries in Dancers." In *Baxter's The Foot and Ankle in Sport*, second edition, edited by David A. Porter and Lew C. Schon, 469–484. Philadelphia, PA: Mosby, Inc.

Omey, Monica L. and Lyle J. Micheli. 1999. "Foot and Ankle Problems in the Young Athlete." *Medicine and Science in Sport and Exercise* 31 (7, July Supplement): S470–S486.

Salonen, D. C., R. Lee, E. J. Becker, A. T. Mascia, and D. Ogilvie-Harris. 1999. "Ankle MR Imaging in the Asymptomatic Dancer." *Abstract 1544, RSNA Annual Meeting.*

Small, Kelly. 2009. "Ankle Sprain and Fractures in Adults." *Orthopaedic Nursing* 28 (6, November/December): 314–320.

Vonhof, John. 2006. *Fixing Your Feet: Prevention and Treatment for Athletes,* fourth edition. Berkeley, CA: Wilderness Press.

10 The Foot

WE NEED OUR FEET TO SERVE AS A PLATFORM FOR STABILITY. CAN YOU IMAGINE IF YOUR TOES WERE ATTACHED RIGHT TO YOUR ANKLE? YOU WOULD JUST TIP RIGHT OVER. NOTHING GRACEFUL ABOUT THAT! FEET HELP CUSHION LANDINGS FROM JETÉ AND HELP POWER OUR JUMPS.

We tend to think that the power of jumps comes from the knees and big thigh muscles. Try seeing how high you can jump, however, using just your knees for power and keeping your foot at a right angle to your leg. You will feel very weak because the foot and ankle muscles help to power the jumps.

FOOT ZONES

Our feet are complex, but we can simplify how we think of them.

If you have pain in your toes or near your toes, it is forefoot pain. Our forefoot includes the front of the foot—metatarsals to toe tips. If you have pain in your arch,

FIG 10-1

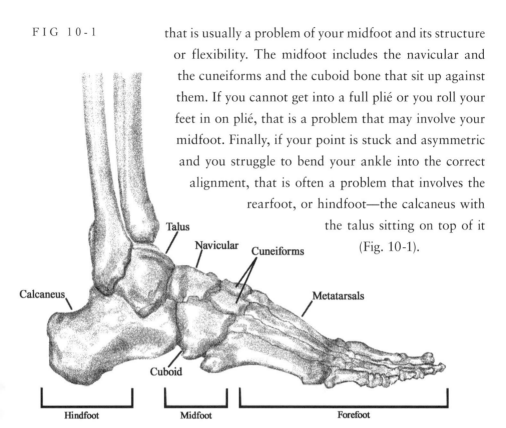

that is usually a problem of your midfoot and its structure or flexibility. The midfoot includes the navicular and the cuneiforms and the cuboid bone that sit up against them. If you cannot get into a full plié or you roll your feet in on plié, that is a problem that may involve your midfoot. Finally, if your point is stuck and asymmetric and you struggle to bend your ankle into the correct alignment, that is often a problem that involves the rearfoot, or hindfoot—the calcaneus with the talus sitting on top of it (Fig. 10-1).

THE FOREFOOT

Our toes attach to our feet and then meet the metatarsals in the front of the foot. The metatarsals are labeled 1 to 5 with the thickest metatarsal of our big toe as number 1. The bump on the outside of the foot is the base of the fifth metatarsal. The balls underneath your feet near your toes are the metatarsal heads (Fig. 10-2). The toes and metatarsals are called the *forefoot*.

FIG 10-2

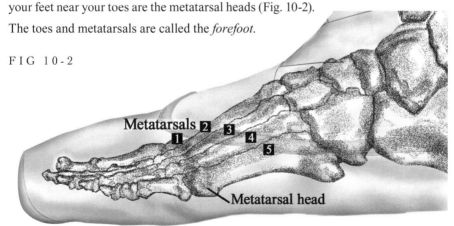

Metatarsal stress fractures

When dancers get stress fractures it is often of these metatarsal bones. Pain in your forefoot that is sharp and localized on the top of your foot may be a metatarsal stress fracture. The most common areas of stress fractures are metatarsals 2 and 3; you will feel pain in your forefoot. If you have tenderness directly over the top of the bone when you point your foot, you probably have a stress fracture and need to rest—or the fracture may become even worse (Fig. 10-3).

FIG 10-3

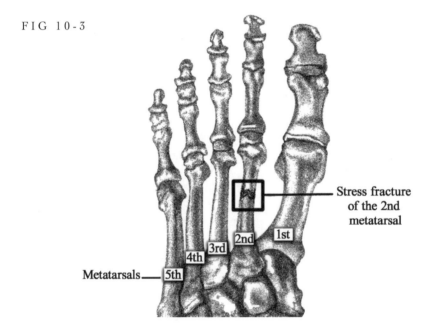

Stress fracture of the 2nd metatarsal

Metatarsals—5th 4th 3rd 2nd 1st

Metatarsal 1 is really thick and mobile so that it is protected against fracture. Metatarsals 4 and 5 are fairly mobile so these bones also can get out of the way and bear less of your weight. Metatarsals 2 and 3 bear a great deal of weight and take a pounding with jumps on a hard floor. Any time you dramatically increase the amount of time in dance class, if you do not have enough calcium in your diet, or if you are not having normal menstrual cycles—you are at higher risk of stress fractures. During Christmastime, when it seems every dance company has *Nutcracker* rehearsals, dancers often receive an additional gift of metatarsal fractures!

MIDFOOT PAIN

The Lisfranc joint

The Lisfranc joint, which is at the base of the second metatarsal (Fig.10-4), is the line where the forefoot meets the midfoot. It is basically directly behind where the metatarsal bones end, near to the ankle. A stress fracture sometimes can be found near the Lisfranc joint. This fracture occurs because metatarsals 1 and 2 take the majority of the force on the foot when it is on demi-pointe or pointe. As the dancer goes on pointe, the second metatarsal is like a strut rigidly locked against the midfoot. So if you are jumping up and down and metatarsal number 2 is correctly locked into place, the base of that second metatarsal takes enormous stress and can fracture.

FIG 10-4

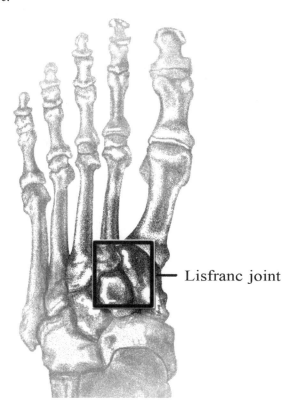

—— Lisfranc joint

If you have unresolving pain in the middle of your foot, you should see your doctor right away because this stress fracture sometimes will not heal correctly if it is not managed properly (Solomon, Solomon, and Minton, ed. 2005, 101).

Dropped metatarsals

Sometimes dancers experience pain directly underneath the metatarsal heads. A metatarsal head can actually drop lower than it supposed to be. This often happens to dancers who perform choreography with a great deal of pointe work or Latin or ballroom dancers who dance in high heels and tight shoes. If you squeeze your forefoot in your hand, you will feel the metatarsal heads drop. The heads of metatarsals 2 and 3 may press against the soft tissue in your foot and get into a dropped position that gives pain.

You can treat this by using a metatarsal pad, which can be found online at Hapad.com. These pads help support the heads of the metatarsal and can give great pain relief (Wheeless 2010).

Locked cuboid

Behind metatarsals 4 and 5 is the cuboid (Fig. 10-5).

FIG 10-5   Cuboid

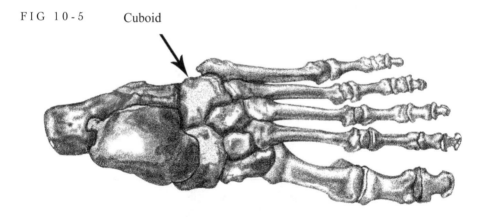

This bone can slip in and out of place in dancers as they go up on pointe. This is called *cuboid subluxation*. The foot will feel weak going onto demi-pointe or pointe and jumps will be painful or difficult, too. This can occur secondary to a dropped or locked cuboid. The cuboid can be placed back into position by a trained physical therapist and then treated with a cuboid pad. Often dancers will sprain an ankle and have residual pain. If an ankle sprain never resolves, you need to be checked for a locked cuboid (Caselli and Pantelaras 2004).

Foot Muscles

The muscles of the foot act as shock absorbers, allow our feet to powerfully propel us into jeté, and stabilize the standing leg.

Muscle weakness

If you find that the toes of your supporting leg are clawing when you stand quietly on one leg, your foot muscles need to be strengthened. The clawing happens because the larger muscles higher up in the leg are trying to compensate for your relatively weak foot muscles. When these larger muscles up the leg overpower your foot muscles, your toes literally begin to claw or curl.

A really good exercise to strengthen your foot muscles is to pull a towel on the floor toward you with your toes. If that is too easy, put a two-to-five pound weight on top of the towel. Also, if you are wobbly when you go up onto pointe, you need to strengthen your foot muscles.

As for muscle pain of the foot, any of the small muscles of the feet can get overworked. If you strengthen your foot muscles, your feet will feel less tired. As an added bonus, if you do foot strengthening exercises, you likely will increase the power of your jumps and decrease the fatigue in your legs.

Flat feet and high-arched feet

The plantar fascia is a tissue band that starts at your inner heel and attaches to your toes. The muscles of the foot along with the *plantar fascia* give us the arch of the foot. If the plantar fascia is torn you get a weak arch or a relatively flat foot. There is a lot of confusion and concern about flatfoot in dance. What is a flat foot, anyway?

Most people develop an arch in their inner foot by age ten. But as many as one out of ten adults never get that arch; they have what is called *flat feet*, or *pes planus* (foot that is flat). A flat foot is, by definition, a more flexible foot. If you walk on paper after your foot is wet and you see the whole print, you have a flat foot. However, if you go on demi-pointe or stand on your toes and your arch magically appears, you have a reversible or flexible flatfoot.

There is no reason you cannot dance with flat feet. As a matter of fact, you may have better shock absorption with your flat feet! However, some people think that flat feet expose you to a greater risk of stress on your low back, so you should do exercises for your core to prevent low back pain secondary to your flat feet.

If you have flat feet and are getting one metatarsal stress fracture after another, you may need to use cushions to redistribute the forces on your feet. One treatment approach to this may be to restore the arch by placing a cuneiform pad under the inner border of the heel that is slightly back from your arch and placing a second pad toward the outside of your foot on the bottom (Wheeless 2009). In addition, dancers with flat feet should also focus on heel cord stretches.

If you have flat feet and have been told (wrongly in my opinion) that it is a problem for dance, do not feel too badly because dancers with high arches also get told they do not have the ideal foot for dance! These dancers may have worse shock absorption than dancers with flat feet, increasing their risk of stress fractures: a high arched foot is a more rigid foot. The shock and stress from dance activity that the beautiful (but poorly shock absorbent), high-arched foot cannot absorb gets distributed to other structures in the foot and cause problems in other areas of the foot (Fig. 10-6).

FIG 10-6

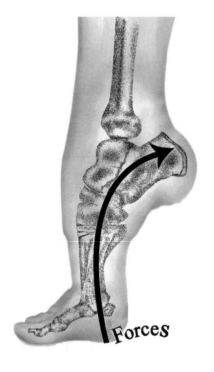
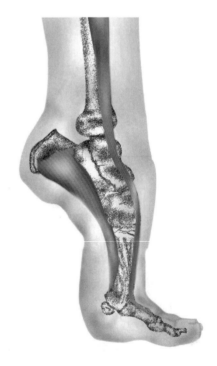

Plantar Fascia and Plantar Fasciitis

The foot has a strap that goes underneath called the *plantar fascia* (Fig. 10-7).

You should think of the plantar fascia as a strap that attaches the base of the toes to the heel base. You can feel the strap of the plantar fascia tighten when the toes go up and the plantar fascia deepens and tightens the arch.

FIG 10-7

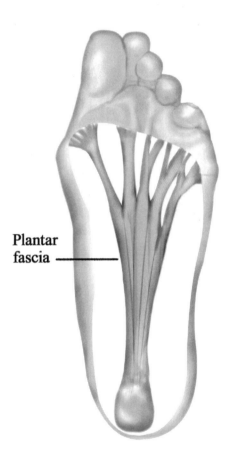

Plantar fascia ————

If you have a really high arch or really low arch or if you are not stretching enough, you can develop plantar fasciitis, tears and pain in the bottom of your foot from inflammation of the plantar fascia. This condition gives you a very painful first step out of bed in the morning, and the rest of the day often does not feel that good either.

It is important to see a doctor if you are a dancer with persistent heel pain because even though you most likely have plantar fasciitis, with pain at the front and inside of your heel, you may have a stress fracture of your heel or a nerve problem. Your doctor can figure that out.

Dancers who have seen a doctor and been told that they have a heel spur have likely had plantar fasciitis badly enough and long enough that a tiny spike of bone has pulled out from where the plantar fascia inserts into your heel (Fig.10-8).

FIG 10-8

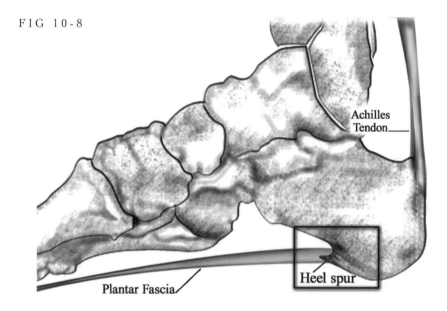

Achilles Tendon

Heel spur

Plantar Fascia

Dance physical therapy helps in treating plantar fasciitis. You will do exercises to strengthen your arch and work on stretching your calf muscles. The Achilles tendon is an extension of the plantar fascia so stretching your plantar fascia and Achilles is important. The Achilles tendon is a thick strap of tissue that is the tendon of your large calf muscles that inserts on the calcaneous. Bringing your foot into dorsiflexion stretches the calf and the Achilles tendon. Remember that your foot flexibility is helped by paying attention to the flexibility of your entire lower leg and calf.

Most plantar fasciitis—approximately 80-90%—will get better by one year without any surgery if the dancer stays focused on stretching (Rompe 2009, 103). Researchers studied what type of stretches work the best and found that pulling up on your toes throughout the day and while pressing the foot arch to ensure that there is a stretch and tension in the plantar fascia was more effective than calf stretches (Fig. 10-9; DiGiovanni et al. 2003, 1274). But I vote that you try both.

FIG 10-9

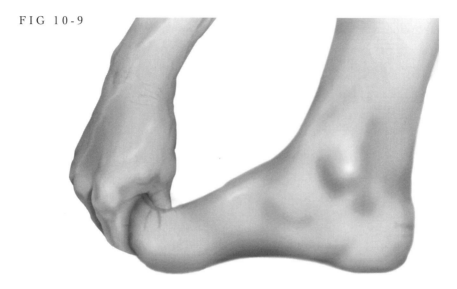

TARSAL TUNNEL SYNDROME

Dancers need to be aware that not all pain on the sole of the foot is plantar fasciitis. There is a nerve called the tibial nerve that goes underneath the arch into the front of your foot and also sends branches back to your heel (Fig. 10-10).

FIG 10-10

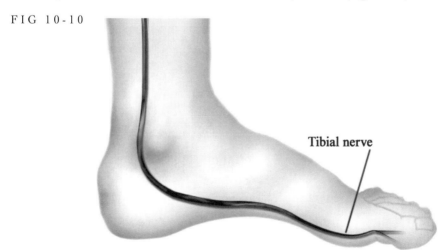

Tibial nerve

Burning and numbness underneath your foot toward your toes and some-times toward your heel can be from injury to this tibial nerve. If you are a dancer who rolls your ankles, you are placing this nerve under traction that can bruise the tibial nerve, causing tarsal tunnel syndrome. Also, dancers who have a large process or bone spur coming off their heel can put pressure on this nerve causing numbness in the foot.

Usually, relieving the pressure and traction on the nerve by using arch strengthening exercises will help with this problem. Dancers with tarsal tunnel syndrome also need to work on calf flexibility.

MORTON'S NEUROMA

Morton's neuroma is a swelling of the nerve between the second and third metatarsals (Fig. 10-11).

FIG 10-11

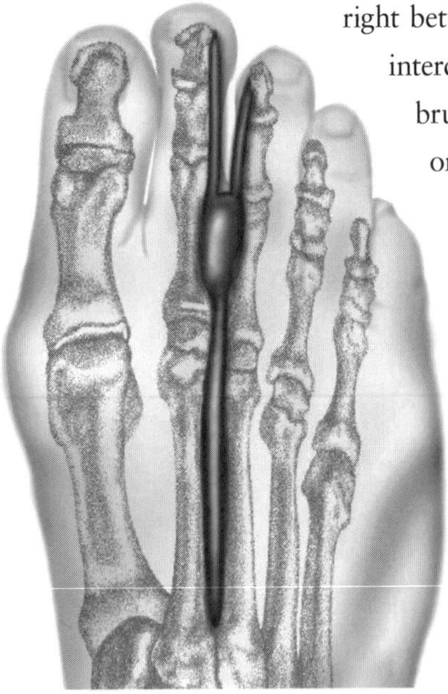

If you feel sort of achy numbness in the front of your foot, right between the second and third metatarsals, your interdigital nerves may be under pressure. Dancers bruise these nerves when they go on demi-pointe or pointe and do jumps. If these nerves get bruised enough, they can develop the swelling called a *Morton's neuroma*. You might feel numbness right between two toes.

If you have a Morton's neuroma, putting a small piece of moleskin or felt just behind the painful area may allow it time to heal as the pressure on the nerve is reduced. You will want to increase the width of your toe box and wear shoes that give your foot more space.

Dancers with numb toes or numb feet need to see a medical doctor as soon as possible! A numb foot can happen because of a serious low back issue or a problem completely separate from your foot. Even if you think you have a neuroma or tarsal tunnel syndrome, be sure to get your foot properly evaluated.

SKIN CONDITIONS

If you have tiny bumps that appear along your foot, these may be piezogenic papules. They often occur near the red/white border of the sole of the foot. They happen because tiny pieces of tissue break through the dermis—probably from repeated trauma, such as dancing. These bumps do not require any specific treatment but cushioning your foot during dance might help (Gebke 2008, 256).

Plantar warts come and go for many dancers. The wart is actually a viral infection that is most often seen on the bottom of the foot (Gebke 2008, 257). If you use over-the-counter medicines for a wart, **please** be sure to follow the directions **exactly**. Some dancers get serious local skin reactions from these products that are more of a problem than the original wart. Even duct tape has been reported to help in the treatment of plantar warts! Try covering your wart with duct tape; leave the tape on about a week; then scrape the wart with an emery board and repeat. If you are diabetic, however, you should let a podiatrist take care of any plantar wart.

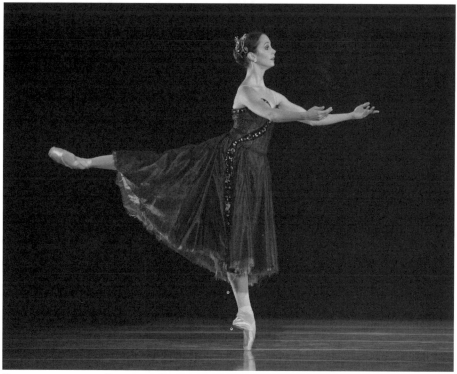

PENNSYLVANIA BALLET PRINCIPAL DANCER JULIE DIANA IN JEROME ROBBINS'S *IN THE NIGHT*. PHOTOGRAPH BY PAUL KOLNIK.

Five Critical Things to Know about Your Feet

1. Anybody with a numb or tingly foot needs to see a medical doctor.

2. If you have pain on the top of your forefoot, you may have a stress fracture and you should get your foot checked by your doctor.

3. Arch pain on the bottom of your foot may be plantar fasciitis—especially likely if your first step in the morning is painful. Exercises and stretches can really help.

4. If you never quite recovered correctly from that ankle sprain, and you have pain toward the outside of your foot, get yourself checked by your doctor and physical therapist. Dancers get lateral foot pain from cuboid problems that can be helped with physical therapy, exercise, and taping.

5. Strong dancers may still have weak feet, and foot exercise will increase your stability and help increase your vertical jump.

Five Foot Exercises and Stretches

1. Crunch your toes together, then fan them apart. Do sets of 10 repetitions.

2. Holding a rail for support, stand on a step with your toes and the balls of your feet on the step and your heels off the step. Slowly rise on both feet and then lower, feeling the stretch in the heel cords. Count to ten in the stretched position and then repeat. Avoid any bouncing with this motion. Do sets of 3-5 repetitions.

3. Using a rubber exercise band, place it around the ball of your foot. Slowly push your foot down against the resistance of the band. You can then loop the band so that you are pulling your foot up against the resistance of the band. This exercise strengthens dorsiflexion and plantarflexion. Do sets of 10 for each foot.

4. Stand on one leg, using a counter for support. Close your eyes and see how long you can balance. Keep repeating this throughout the day.

5. While you are seated, put a towel on the floor and pull it toward you with your toes; then push it away. Do 5–10 repetitions.

References

Caselli, Mark A., DPM, and Nikiforos Pantelaras, DPM. 2004. "How to Treat Cuboid Syndrome in the Athlete." *Podiatry Today* 17 (10, October 1): 76–80.

Digiovanni, Benedict F., MD, Deborah A. Nawoczenski, PhD, PT, Daniel P. Malay, MSPT, Petra A. Graci, DPT, Taryn T. Williams, MSPT, Gregory E. Wilding, PhD, and Judith F. Baumhauer, MD. 2006. "Plantar Fascia—Specific Stretching Exercise Improves Outcomes in Patients with Chronic Plantar Fasciitis." *The Journal of Bone and Joint Surgery* (American) 88 (8): 1775–1781.

DiGiovanni, Benedict F., MD, Deborah A. Nawoczenski, PhD PT, Marc E. Lintal, MS, PT, Elizabeth A. Moore, MS, PT, Joseph C. Murray, MS, PT, Gregory E. Wilding, PhD, and Judith F. Baumhauer, MD. 2003. "Tissue-Specific Plantar Fascia Stretching Exercise Enhances Outcomes in Patients with Chronic Heel Pain." *The Journal of Bone and Joint Surgery* 85 (7): 1270–1277.

Gebke, Kevin. "Dermatologic, Infectious, and Nail Disorders." 2008. In *Baxter's The Foot and Ankle in Sport*, second edition, edited by David A. Porter and Lew C. Schon, 251–259. Philadelphia, PA: Mosby, Inc.

Kennedy, John G., Chistopher W. Hodgkins, Jean-Alain Columbier, and William G. Hamilton. 2008. "Foot and Ankle Injuries in Dancers." In *Baxter's The Foot and Ankle in Sport*, second edition, edited by David A. Porter and Lew C. Schon, 469–484. Philadelphia, PA: Mosby, Inc.

Omey, Monica L. and Lyle J. Micheli. 1999. "Foot and Ankle Problems in the Young Athlete." *Medicine and Science in Sports and Exercise* 31 (7, July Supplement): S470–S486.

Rompe, Jan D. 2009. "Plantar Fasciopathy." *Sports Medicine and Arthroscopy Review* 17 (2): 100–104.

Solomon, Ruth, John Solomon, and Sandra Cerny Minton, editors. 2005. *Preventing Dance Injuries,* second edition. Champaign, IL: Human Kinetics.

Stretanski, Michael F. and G. J. Weber. 2002. "Medical and Rehabilitation Issues in Classical Ballet: Literature Review." *American Journal of Physical Medicine and Rehabilitation* 81 (5): 383–391.

Wheeless, Clifford R., III. 2009. "Pes Planus/Flat Foot." *Wheeless' Textbook of Orthopaedics.* Last update February 4. http://www.wheelessonline.com/ortho/pes_planus_flat_foot.

———. 2010. "Orthotics for the Foot." *Wheeless' Textbook of Orthopaedics.* Last update July 25. http://www.wheelessonline.com/ortho/orthotics_for_the_foot.

11 The Toes

W E NEED TOES TO HELP US WITH BALANCE AND TO INCREASE
THE LENGTH OF THE FOOT. TOES PROVIDE
POWER FOR JUMPS AND HELP
ABSORB THE SHOCK OF LANDINGS. THERE
ARE, OF COURSE, FIVE TOES ON EACH
FOOT. THE TOES ARE NUMBERED ONE
TO FIVE STARTING FROM THE INSIDE
OF THE FOOT TOWARD THE ARCH AND
WORKING TOWARD THE OUTSIDE. THE
BIG TOE IS CALLED THE *HALLUX*
AND THE FIFTH TOE IS THE
BABY TOE (FIG. 11-1).

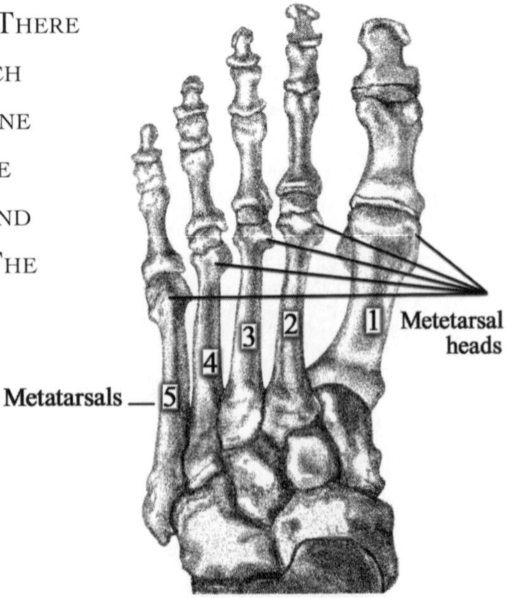

Metetarsal
heads

Metatarsals

FIG 11-1

Bones of the Toes

Generally speaking, the toes are arranged as an arc in terms of their length. The big toe, or hallux, has one joint; the other toes each have two joints. (A stubbed toe is usually an injury to one of those joints.) The bones of all of the toes are called the *phalanges*. The toes then abut the heads of the metatarsal bones, the bones that are those toward the front of the foot (Fig. 11-2).

FIG 11-2

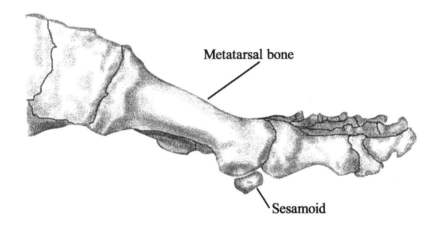

Metatarsal bone

Sesamoid

Additional tiny bones called the *sesamoids* lie underneath the big toe and act like force dispersing shock absorbers. Each big toe has two small sesamoids. Surprisingly, fifty percent of the weight carried by each foot is carried by the hallux (big toe), which can support all of this weight because it is so thick and because it has this special feature, the sesamoid bones. These tiny bones, about the size of sesame seeds, slide underneath the big toe when the big toe moves.

Muscles that Move the Toes

Toes can move because muscles attach to the toes via the tendons. The *flexor hallucis longus* muscle is what moves the big toe down toward the floor and gives you power to get up on pointe. The flexor hallucis longus and the *flexor digitorum longus* muscle pull the toe down when they contract and this gives the foot the ability to point (Fig. 11-3). The pulling action of these two muscles also increases the stretch on the top of the foot.

FIG 11-3

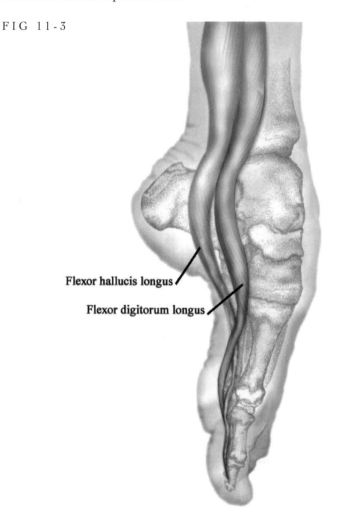

Flexor hallucis longus

Flexor digitorum longus

TOE INJURIES
Tendonitis of the flexor hallucis longus

To achieve a beautiful point, dancers may overstress the flexor hallucis longus muscle and it can develop a painful swelling, causing the big toe to stick and trigger. If your big toe is sticking and there is pain behind your inner ankle, you may have developed tendonitis of the flexor hallucis longus, the tendon that attaches to the hallux. A physical therapist can help this by ultrasound and stretching treatment.

Your alignment and technique can be part of the problem and a dance physical therapist can help to correct this condition early. If the condition is allowed to become too severe, you may need surgery to free the tendon. Do not delay seeing a doctor if your toe is sticking or triggering! Correct physical therapy may spare you a surgery that likely will knock you out for a season.

Range of motion issues

Classical ballet certainly demands a great deal of the big toe! The range of motion needed to achieve a good demi-pointe and pointe is extreme: a successful demi-pointe relevé requires 90 degrees of dorsiflexion. In other words, your toe needs to go up to a right angle to your foot if you do not want to stress the rest of your foot to get that nice position.

Because dancers always want to push to the extreme, the great toe joint gets banged up all the time. Any joint that gets a great deal of use can undergo degeneration. The degeneration leads to the development of bone spurs around the joint. These bone spurs make the joint feel stiff, so then the dancer forces the range even more and the toe gets stiffer yet!

Hallux rigidis: a stiff big toe

If you see a bump on the top of your big toe, and if your toe feels like it is stiffening, you may be developing what is called *hallux rigidus*, or "stiff big toe," in medical terms. If you do have this stiff toe, gentle traction on the toe will relax the muscles and help you with your range of motion. Use a foot whirlpool, too.

Consider working with a physical therapist to see if work on the soft tissues of the big toe will get back sufficient range of motion. In phonophoresis, a trained clinician uses an ultrasound machine to drive anti-inflammatory medicine through your skin to the sore area. This technique can be very helpful. Sometimes though, those bone spurs will have to be removed. An orthopedist or foot doctor actually has to shave the tiny bone spurs so the joint can get through enough range of motion to achieve correct positioning.

Hallux length and Morton's toe

The length of the hallux matters, too. Dr. Kadel and other researchers looked at the ratio of the length of the second metatarsal to the first to determine if a relatively short first toe caused problems in dance. They found that if the first metatarsal was shorter by even about 20% then dancers developed more arthritis of the arch area, which is terrible for a dancer because it causes all kinds of problems working through the foot.

And there is more: some dancers have an overly long second toe called a Morton's toe (no relationship to the Morton's neuroma condition, discussed in Chapter 10) (Fig. 11-4).

Ideally, your toes are about the same length giving you a wide base of support for the actions of your foot and leg. Dancers with a Morton's toe will experi-

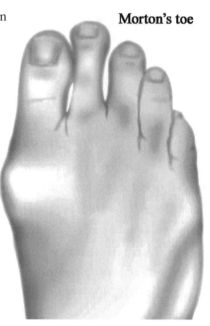

Morton's toe

FIG 11-4

ence issues going on pointe. The long second toe takes too much of the pressure. Therefore, if you have a relatively long second toe, you will want to think about padding your big toe in the pointe shoe so the forces are better distributed in the shoe block. Dancers with a long second toe can purchase pads from Hapad (available at Hapad.com) or use lamb's wool padding in the pointe shoe block.

Sesamoiditis

Unfortunately, the tiny sesamoid bones (which are under the big toe) are subject to injury. The sesamoid toward the inside part of your foot is usually the one that is injured. There will be a lot of pain with walking or jumping, and also tenderness directly underneath the ball of the foot.

I have seen many dancers with pain underneath the first toe. Often, it seems to be in younger dancers who are first beginning to go up on pointe. Sesamoiditis is an inflammation of these bones. Classical dancers are often bruising sesamoids secondary to bad landings from jumps. Demi-pointe puts direct pressure on the sesamoids and they can become inflamed from extensive demi-pointe work. If the dancer's hallux angles inward, the sesamoids are more exposed, which increases the trauma to the sesamoids as well.

Sesamoids can be treated by taping and resting from demi-pointe.

If you have persistent pain underneath your toe that does not respond to rest, a doctor needs to check your toe to make sure that the sesamoids have not fractured. A sesamoid fracture can occur secondary to a sudden jump or even repetitive stress.

Turf toe

Underneath the big toe, the capsule that contains the sesamoids can also become injured. If your big toe is suddenly flexed up, say in a bad landing from a jump, or you fall off your demi-pointe to the inside, you can tear this capsule. A tear of this capsule, called *turf toe*, causes pain underneath the first toe (Hockenberry 1999). This pain is right in the ball of the foot at the base of the hallux (Fig. 11-5).

FIG 11-5

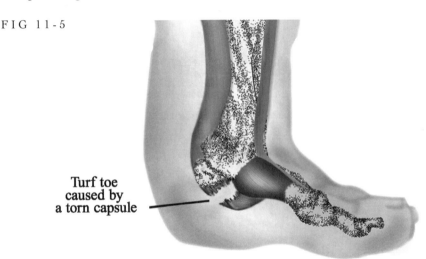

Turf toe
caused by
a torn capsule

If you think you have a turf toe, it is important to be seen by a physician because turf toe injuries can be very serious. If you have injured this capsule, your doctor will most likely recommend a period of rest followed by splinting the toe. Carbon graphite splints are specific to turf toe and stabilize the foot during activity so the capsule is less likely to be torn again. Relevé and pointe work are very difficult for most dancers to return to after a capsule injury to the hallux base. I suggest that any dancer who has a turf toe injury work with a physical therapist experienced in dance to regain their stability in relevé and pointe work. The big toe flexor will need to be restrengthened.

Two exercises that help toe strength are putting a towel on the floor and crunching it up with your toes and placing small marbles on the floor and picking them up with your toes. As you heal from a turf toe injury, you will need to work on the following toe fanning exercise: sit and spread the toes into a fan, then release. This will tend to relax the tightness in the foot that you get as the turf toe heals.

Bunions

If your big toe looks like it is drifting at an angle you are likely developing a bunion (Fig. 11-6).

FIG 11-6

 Bunion ___

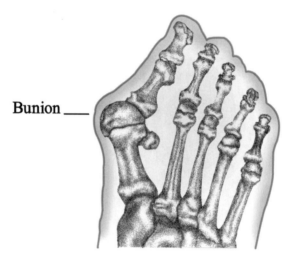

Bunions are very common in dancers. Actually they are common, period. (Hart, deAsla, and Grottkau 2008, 274).

Going up on pointe, wearing tight shoes, and wearing shoes that do not fit correctly do not necessarily cause bunions but they certainly do not help your feet. Injury to the joint of the big toe may predispose a dancer to the eventual development of hallux valgus, or bunion (Schon 2009, 84). Also, a relatively short first metatarsal ray, the relatively large bone that goes to the base of the big toe, a relatively tight gastroc-soleus muscle, hypermobility of your foot and hyperpronation all contribute (Fig. 11-7; Davitt et al. 2005, 799).

Dancers who tend to have a weak arch often put extra pressure on the hallux, which will contribute to the formation of a bunion. Women are much more

FIG 11-7

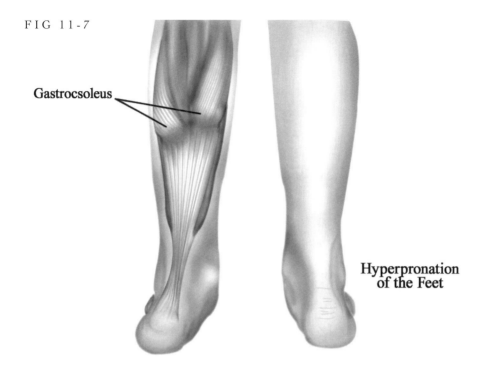

Gastrocsoleus

Hyperpronation of the Feet

frequently affected by bunions than men and there is some tendency for bunions to run in families. The most important thing to know about bunions in dancers is that, generally, bunions should not be treated surgically. Surgery can result in permanent stiffness, which, in a dancer, is catastrophic and potentially career-ending. The complication rate of bunion surgery has reported to be 10% to around–50%! Please do not let this be you!

If the superficial bump on your bunion is irritated, place a small piece of moleskin over the bump. There are also bunion pads that can be directly placed on the bunion. You can purchase these pads from Hapad, Inc. (at www.hapad.com) and FootSmart (at www.footsmart.com). Engo® performance patches, lightweight patches that can be attached to your pointe shoe, can be helpful (available at www.goengo.com). These products can be really great at reducing some of the irritation at the bump.

Do not forget the obvious and adjust your pointe shoe to a wider toe box shoe. In addition, place a small pad between the first and second toes and to see if that helps decrease the stress on the first metatarsophalangeal joint.

Corns, calluses, and blisters

If you have pain between your toes, you might be developing corns. Corns, a pressure and sweat phenomenon commonly seen in dancers' feet, can be hard or soft but they all hurt. A corn is just that, a kernel of thick skin that builds up with pressure—waxy looking yellow bumps.

If you need to soften a corn, Epsom salt soaks and warm water baths are helpful. Any area with pressure should ideally be padded with moleskin or lamb's wool. Soft corns in between the toes are worsened by sweat so try to wear cotton or wick socks when you are not dancing, and put paper towels between the toes and change them often.

You also may have calluses on your toes. Calluses are typically on the bottom of your toes (and your heels, and your forefoot near the toes under the balls of the toes). Calluses need to be treated with the respect they deserve because they are your stripes as a dancer showing that you have done your time to beat your feet up enough to have tough dry skin on your feet. Calluses protect you and should not be removed without a good reason. If they are getting too big and interfering, however, soak you foot and apply moisturizing lotion. Take a pumice stone and gently remove the least amount of callus you can so that your foot remains protected (Shah 2008, 131).

If you are dancing on your blisters instead of your feet use Bodyglide® Anti-chafe, Vaseline®, or even ChapStick® to decrease the friction. Do not unroof or pop blisters. If your blister is bigger than your foot and you simply must (although I would advise you to resist temptation), use sterile equipment and just prick the blister enough to get under the roof and let it drain; then cover it with a protective bandage. Moleskin or felt also can be used in shoes as protection.

Finally, if your toes are cracked and bleeding seal them for performance with liquid Band-aids® and treat them with topical antibiotics.

Numbness between two toes is often associated with a nerve problem higher up in the foot from a swelling called a Morton's *neuroma* (see page 132).

A painful bump on digit five, the baby toe, is called a *bunionette* (Fig.11-8).

Bunion pads work great on bunionettes. Gently stretch your toes at night to relax the muscles of the foot near the bunionette and, by all means, stabilize your bunionette with a tiny pad in between toes 4 and 5. Again, keep away from surgery if at all possible.

FIG 11-8

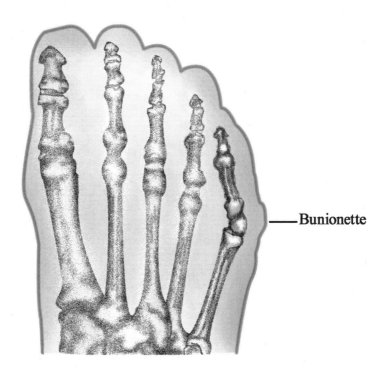

———Bunionette

POINTE SHOES

The search for the right pointe shoe can be a frustrating journey for many ballet dancers. Seek the advice of your dance teacher and try different shoes. Remember that as you train, your needs in a pointe shoe may change. Listen to your feet and to your teacher! Do not use shoes that squeeze your toes too tightly together or that allow you to slide around (Reinhardt 2008, 25).

FINAL THOUGHTS—THE FLOOR

Dancers often dance on a floor that is called a *Marley* floor or a semi-sprung floor. These dance floors are specially designed to help cushion landings and give some energy back to the dancer as the dancer moves about on the floor. They are very important to the health of dancers. Dancers who dance on concrete or a tile or non-spring surface greatly increase their risk of overuse injuries and stress fractures. Check your studio! If you are dancing on a concrete slab that has not been modified, dance yourself right out the front door.

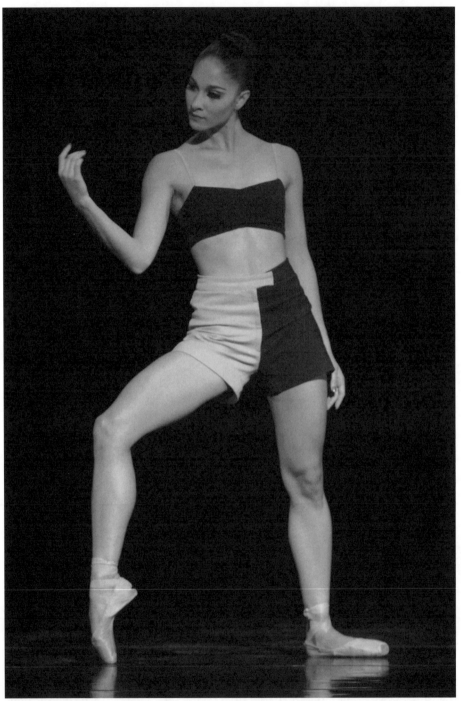

PENNSYLVANIA BALLET SOLOIST GABRIELLA YUDENICH IN MAURO BIGONZETTI'S
KAZIMIR'S COLOURS. PHOTOGRAPH BY PAUL KOLNIK.

The Dancer's Abbreviated Guide to Toes: Could it be This?

1. Pain at outside of big toe, toe slanting in: could be the start of a bunion.

2. Pain at top of big toe: could be the start of hallux rigidus, could be an inflammatory arthritic condition, such as gout.

3. Pain underneath big toe: could be sesamoiditis or turf toe.

4. Pain at end of second toe when you are on pointe: could be a Morton's toe.

5. Pain in between toes with swelling: could be a corn or blister.

6. Numbness in between toes—likely Morton's neuroma. (See Chapter 10.)

7. Nail growing into the soft part of toe: ingrown toenail.

8. Pain at outside of baby toe: could be a bunionette starting.

9. Big toe is snapping or triggering to get through range of motion—trigger toe: likely associated with chronic flexor hallucis longus tendonitis.

The Five Key Toe Tips to Help the Dancer

1. Think very carefully before trimming any calluses on your toes. Those calluses protect your toes.

2. Bunion surgery is an option of very last resort since it can lead to permanent stiffness of the toe and may be career-ending surgery for a dancer.

3. If your toes are cramping and tight at night, gentle stretching or items such as yoga socks will help. However if you are gripping too much with your toes, you might have a problem with your balance. You should get yourself evaluated by your teacher and a dance medicine practitioner to see what can be done to help your placement.

4. Be very careful that your pointe shoes fit. If you are wearing them until they are just a cardboard tatter of a toe box or until your toes are so tight in them that they are wedged, you are both limiting your ability to show off your skill as a dancer and exposing your legs to injury.

5. If you have bunion pain, think about a pointe shoe (and a street shoe) with a wider toe box. Also consider using a pad in between your first and second toes to assist with positioning.

References

Clippinger, Karen Sue. 2007. *Dance Anatomy and Kinesiology*. Champaign, IL: Human Kinetics.

Davitt, James S., MD, Nancy Kadel, MD, Bruce J. Sangeorzan, MD, Sigvard T. Hansen, Jr., MD, Sarah K. Holt, MPH, and Emily Donaldson-Fletcher, BA. 2005. "An Association Between Functional Second Metatarsal Length and Midfoot Arthrosis." *The Journal of Bone and Joint Surgery (American)* 87 (4, April): 795–800.

Fitt, Sally Sevey. 1996. *Dance Kinesiology*, second edition. New York: Schirmer Books.

Hart, Erin S., Richard J. deAsla, and Brian E. Grottkau. 2008. "Current Concepts in the Treatment of Hallux Valgus." *Orthopedic Nursing* 27 (5, September/October): 274–280.

Hockenbury, R. Todd. 1999. "Forefoot Problems in Athletes." *Medicine and Science in Sports and Exercise* 31 (7, July Supplement): S448–S458.

Mann, Roger. 2008. "Bunion Deformity in Elite Athletes." In *Baxter's The Foot and Ankle in Sport*, second edition, edited by David A. Porter and Lew C. Schon, 435–444. Philadelphia, PA: Mosby, Inc.

McMinn, Robert M. H., Ralph T. Hutchings, and Bari M. Logan. 1996. *Color Atlas of Foot and Ankle Anatomy*, second edition. London, UK: Mosby-Wolfe.

Meloã, Lina, Miguel Castro, Lina Chen, Tudor Hughes, and Donald Resnick. 2009. "Differential Diagnosis of Nonneoplastic Forefoot Pain." *Contemporary Diagnostic Radiology* 32 (6): 1–5.

Reinhardt, Angela. 2008. *Pointe Shoes: Tips and Tricks for Choosing, Tuning, Care*. Alton, Hampshire, UK: Dance Books Ltd.

Schon, Lew C. 2009. "Assessment of the Foot and Ankle in Elite Athletes." *Sports Medicine and Arthroscopy Review* 17 (2): 82–86.

Shah, Selina. 2008. "Caring for the Dancer: Special Considerations for the Performer and Troupe." *Current Sports Medicine Reports 7 (3, May/June): 128–132.*

Vonhof, John. 2006. *Fixing Your Feet: Prevention and Treatment for Athletes*, fourth edition. Berkeley, CA: Wilderness Press.

12 Optimizing Performance for a Lifetime

I Want to Dance Forever

P HYSIOLOGY IS THE STUDY OF HOW YOUR BODY FUNCTIONS
TO MAINTAIN ITSELF. DANCE EXERCISE PHYSIOLOGY IS THE
SCIENCE OF DEVELOPING YOUR PHYSICAL ABILITY TO FUNCTION
AS A DANCER — YOUR ABILITY TO DEVELOP HIGH SPEED, ENDURANCE,
AND PRECISION IN ALL OF YOUR MOVEMENTS. YOUR ABILITY TO RISE TO
DIFFERENT DEMANDS, SUCH AS HOLDING A STILL POSE OR DOING A LEAP
INTO THE AIR, IS THE CRITICAL PHYSICAL BASIS OF YOUR ABILITY TO DANCE.

ALL DANCERS SHOULD HAVE A BASIC UNDERSTANDING OF HOW DANCE
HAPPENS.

AEROBIC EXERCISE

A brief burst of energy, such as for a leap, uses anaerobic energy. *Anaerobic*
means *without oxygen*. Your endurance, however, is based on aerobic fitness.
Aerobic exercise means muscles use oxygen to contract and work. Oxygen gets
to muscles because the heart pumps blood rich in oxygen to the muscles. In

addition, skeletal muscle has slow twitch fibers and fast twitch fibers. Slow twitch, or red, fibers use oxygen and can sustain long-duration activities. Fast twitch, or white, fibers can contract very rapidly but only for a brief burst of activity. The slow twitch muscle fibers are used in endurance activities. When you have good endurance, you do not gasp for air after you have made one sweep across the dance studio. To have good aerobic capacity and to have great endurance in dance and all athletics, you need a good aerobic capacity and a strong heart and lungs.

Dancers do not get perfectly aerobically trained by dance. Center floor exercises are too brief and too interrupted. Dancers are weaker than other athletes and can improve their strength through training. You cannot simply stretch and dance. You also need to aerobically train and exercise to be the best dancer you can be.

THE MYTH OF THE DANCER'S PERFECT BODY

No dancer has a perfect body. All dancers have subtle asymmetries. But dancers can be very good at perfecting how they **use** their bodies to achieve artistry in dance.

Dancers can use dance screenings as a tool to get more information about their movement patterns and asymmetries to correct faults and improve technique. These screenings, done by a variety of dance medicine clinicians, usually evaluate your overall health and conditioning and also examine for range of motion asymmetries or strength deficits. This information can help guide your conditioning program (Potter et al. 2008).

That being said, dancers do exhibit a fairly consistent body composition throughout their performance careers. Researchers had noted that professional female ballet dancers' body fat ranged from 14% to 19% (Twitchett, Koutedakis, and Wyon 2009, 2735). Female dancers in an elite professional college program have been studied as well. The average body fat percentage again was approximately 19% (Yannakoulia 2000, 230).

Although you might think that all of the dance training makes you strong, many dancers have muscular strength imbalances. For example, a dancer may have a stronger knee extensor than a knee flexor. These imbalances predispose the dancer to injury.

CARDIOVASCULAR CONDITIONING

Cardiovascular conditioning is important for all of us. It is true that dancers spend hours and hours exercising, but ballet and dance are not great cardiovascular conditioning exercises (Twitchett 2009, 2733). Aerobic exercise is needed to exercise your heart effectively. This means that your heart needs at least 15 minutes of exercising at a rapid rate in order to be exercised—a rate of about sixty percent of your predicted maximum heart rate. Dance class provides, at best, moderate aerobic exercise. As a result, ballet and modern dancers need to do additional exercise for their hearts so that they will have good endurance in class. Part of dancing forever is having a heart that is healthy. What type of endurance exercise should you do? Swimming, bike riding, fast walking, hiking—all are perfectly OK. Just monitor your heart rate so you get the conditioning that you need.

Target heart rate

It is very easy to figure out your target heart rate. Just do 220 minus your age in years. So, for example, if you are eighteen years old, 220 − 18 = 202. Now multiply that by 0.6, and that's it. If you are eighteen years old, you multiply 202 x 0.6 = 121.2. That is the target heart or pulse rate you should reach when you do your aerobic training.

To check your pulse, take the middle three fingers of your left hand, put them on your right wrist and press until you feel your radial pulse. Measure your pulse for six seconds and multiply by ten. That is how fast your heart is beating, as long as your pulse is regular. (If your pulse is not regular, go get yourself checked by a doctor!)

Now that you know the formula above, start thinking about your training. There are many different formulas that are used to calculate a target heart rate. But the principle is very simple: if you do not exercise your heart, it will not get stronger and more effective at pumping blood to muscle and you will fatigue more quickly.

SOME THOUGHTS ON EXERCISES FOR STRENGTH, ENDURANCE, AND FLEXIBILITY IN DANCE

Exercise to improve your endurance should be done most days. The Centers for Disease Control now recommends that at least two-and-a-half hours (150 minutes) of moderate-intensity aerobic activity, such as brisk walking or biking, be done every week by adults. For most people that translates into exercising most days of the week to get in the aerobic exercise needed to stay heart healthy. In addition, an adult should do strengthening activities that work the arms, chest, back, and legs at least twice a week. You can do this exercise with resistance bands, free weights, or machines (Centers for Disease Control and Prevention 2010).

Dancers also need to do exercises specific to dance. Lifting a twenty-pound barbell fifty times will not do one thing to improve the look of your press lift as a dancer. Doing a workout of hamstring curls on a machine at the gym will not do one thing to improve the look of your plié. Your exercise needs to be specific to dance.

Eric Franklin has written extensively on the topic of dance-specific conditioning. Your exercise should be tailored to what you need to do in dance. Training and conditioning for dancers is very different from the training and conditioning of a long-distance runner. Your training for dance needs to focus on speed, balance, range of motion, and flexibility.

Warm-up

All dancers should warm up before conditioning. Warming up allows blood to go to muscles and to tendons to relax and stretch them (Franklin 2004, 9–11). Three minutes of light running in place should do the trick. You need to literally "warm up." Your body actually should feel slightly warmer to you when you are finished.

Start concentrating on how your body feels during the warm-up. You are doing an activity to prepare your body. Pay attention to how your body is feeling. If you feel shoulder tightness or your left hamstring feels tighter than the right, these are the areas that are going to limit your workout. Stretch these areas; spend extra time and think carefully about how your body is responding.

Mind/body conditioning

Next, lighten up your mind to loosen up your muscles. Let go of stress; the muscles then relax, too. A relaxed muscle can quickly adapt to balance challenges.

Eric Franklin talks about simple weight shifts to get your mind and body attuned. Try standing in parallel, shift one foot forward, see how this feels, and shift back. Try this again with your eyes closed and feel the difference. Do the exercise again, shifting your feet with your eyes open and then your eyes closed while lifting your arms over your head. Do the exercise again while music is playing on your left. Move the music source to your right. Feel how your body responds to all of these different challenges. Your visual field, the lighting of the floor, the hardness of the floor, the direction of the music, your footwear—all of these factors and more come into play and affect your balance when you are trying to dance.

Positive psychology and dance

Because dancers are surrounded by people commenting on how they are doing, dancers need to maintain a positive internal balance. Try to make your thinking positive about yourself so that you allow yourself to improve. Dancers need balance in mind as well as in body to perform. Instead of expecting failure, internally plan for success. This is a more helpful approach. Dancers have disciplined bodies; dancers also need to focus on discipling their thoughts. Each dance class is another opportunity to put positive psychology in place so that you can improve as a dancer (Branner and Branner 2007, 54-55; Hamilton and New York City Ballet 2008, 146-147).

MOTOR LEARNING AND MUSCLE MEMORY
Chunking

When you see dance on the stage it appears to be effortless. It flows.

The muscles have a memory of the patterns of the dance. When dancers spend long hours in class and repeat the linked steps over and over again, the brain and nerves become more and more efficient at making that movement pattern happen without conscious thought. Just as your muscles remember how to ride a bicycle, your muscles will begin to remember the dance movements that you repeat over and over (Solway 2007).

This nerve learning of the individual components of a dance so that it is hardwired into your brain and then automatically performed by your muscles is called *chunking*. When your muscles have the memory, you are not stiff, movement is smooth, and your brain is freed up to concentrate on the artistry of the dance performance.

Muscle memory can even start with watching the movement patterns. This means that even if you have an injury and you cannot perform, you should try to get to class. Your attention to the movements gets your brain thinking about the patterns. When you can start to move again, this attentive watching may be helpful to develop the muscle memory that you need.

SETTING REALISTIC GOALS

If we set goals for ourselves on how we want to move and dance, we can improve and feel good about what is happening in class. But if our goals are unrealistic, we cannot possibly succeed in achieving them.

It is important to be able to set realistic goals in dance. First, think carefully about what you want to achieve in dance. If you want to dance to have fun, great! Then make sure that dance **is** fun—that you do not get injured by doing routines that are technically beyond your abilities. If your goal is to major in dance or dance professionally, then set goals that you can reach. For example, instead of saying, "I will have a perfect class and the teacher will use **me** as the example for all the others," focus on, "I will be able to smoothly do the allegro sequence today." Think carefully about what is in that one dance sequence, visualize the sequence, be warmed up, stretched, and ready. Do your practice visualization. Do your motor repetitions of the movement to get muscle memory, and conquer the sequence so that you succeed. Break your dance sequences down into shorter segments that you can master—then try to combine those sequences.

Goals can be even more specific. For example, you can practice standing on one leg with your arms stretched out and have a goal of standing ten seconds longer without having to touch down the other foot. Then practice, practice, practice. With practice, you will succeed. And then you can progress to additional goals (Hamilton 1998, 136-137).

Part of setting reasonable goals is giving yourself a reasonable time frame in which to achieve them. Muscle memory, performance ease, and grace in dance all take time. The effortless performance on stage is built on the small steps of practice and setting achievable goals along the way.

I WANT TO DANCE FOREVER

I want you to dance forever. You want you to dance forever. A positive approach to your health and dancing will take you a long way toward this goal. This book is really the start of the lifetime of dance ahead of you. Keep your goal of a lifetime of dance at the top of your mind in each class.

If you think about dancing for your lifetime—not just surviving one tough class—you will be well on your way to your healthy lifetime of dance (Potter et al. 2008). Remember to work on disciplining your thoughts and your body.

Exercise your heart and lungs and not just your legs and arms! Take charge and take care of mental and physical well-being. Pay attention to any injuries and promptly get yourself the help you need. And remember, balance in all things in life (not just in dance)!

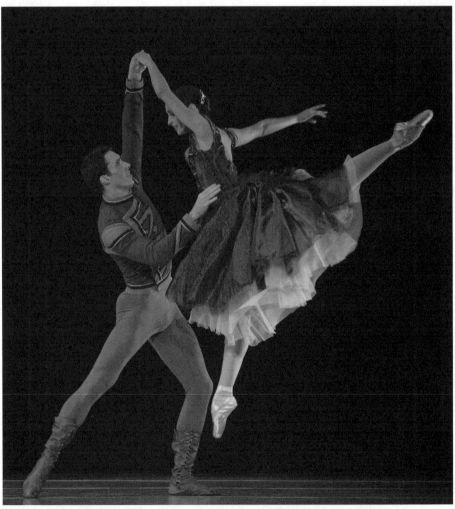

PENNSYLVANIA BALLET PRINCIPAL DANCER RIOLAMA LORENZO AND SOLOIST JAMES IHDE IN JEROME ROBBINS'S *IN THE NIGHT*. PHOTOGRAPH BY PAUL KOLNIK.

References

Branner, Toni Tickel and Jenna Lee Branner. 2007. *The Care and Feeding of a Dancer: What You Need to Know On and Off the Stage.* Waxhaw, NC: Blue Water Press.

Centers for Disease Control and Prevention: Division of Nutrition, Physical Activity, and Obesity, National Center for Chronic Disease Prevention and Health Promotion. 2010. "Physical Activity for Everyone: How much physical activity do you need?" Last updated August 30. http://www.cdc.gov/physicalactivity/everyone/guidelines.

Franklin, Eric. 2004. *Conditioning for Dance: Training for Peak Performance in All Dance Forms.* Champaign, IL: Human Kinetics.

Hamilton, Linda H. 1998. *Advice for Dancers: Emotional Counsel and Practical Strategies.* San Francisco: Jossey-Bass Inc., Publishers.

Hamilton, Linda H. and New York City Ballet. 2008. *The Dancer's Way: The New York City Ballet Guide to Mind, Body, and Nutrition.* New York: St. Martin's Griffin.

Koutedakis, Yiannis. 2001. "Physiological Aspects of Dance." In *Sports Medicine for Specific Ages and Abilities,* edited by Nicola Maffulli, Kai Ming Chan, Rose Macdonald, Robert M. Malina, and Anthony W. Parker, 187–194. London, UK: Churchill Livingston.

Nordin, Margareta and Victor H. Frankel. 2001. *Basic Biomechanics of the Musculoskeletal System,* third edition. Baltimore, MD: Lippincott Williams and Wilkins.

Potter, Karen, Marliese Kimmerle, Gayanne Grossman, Margot Rijven, Marijeanne Liederbach, and Virginia Wilmerding. 2008. "Screening in a Dance Wellness Program." Education Committee and Research Committee, International Association for Dance Medicine and Science.

Solway, Diane. 2007. "Learning to Dance, One Chunk at a Time." *The New York Times*, May 27.

Twitchett, Emily A., Yiannis Koutedakis, and Matthew A. Wyon. 2009. "Physiological Fitness and Professional Classical Ballet Performance: A Brief Review." [Review] *The Journal of Strength and Conditioning Research.* 23 (9, December): 2732–2740.

Yannakoulia, Mary, Antonios Keramopoulos, Nikolaos Tsakalakos, and Antonia-Leda Matalas. 2000. "Body composition in dancers: the bioelectrical impedance method." *Medicine & Science in Sports & Exercise.* 32(1, January): 228-234.

Dancer Resources

FIVE HELPFUL WEBSITES (PLUS ONE!)

http://www.med.nyu.edu/hjd/harkness

The Harkness Center for Dance Injuries is in New York City. The website has some thoughts and information on common dance injuries. Some financial aid for injured dancers is offered and some services for dancers are subsidized.

www.iadms.org

This is the website of the International Association of Dance Medicine and Science. You will find very helpful consensus papers here that have been prepared by panels with experts who are familiar with the dance world. The papers range in topic from thoughts on when to first consider going on pointe to nutritional advice for the dancer and dance student.

www.dance-teacher.com

The website of *Dance Teacher* magazine: a great resource for teachers and students, with helpful articles for all dancers who are either beginning or established in their careers.

www.dancemagazine.com

The website of *Dance Magazine*. Gorgeous photography. Cool videos of dancers. Fantastic articles. In my opinion, the college guide is particularly helpful. This list alone makes *Dance Magazine* worth your time. Purchase a subscription and scan the site, too.

www.renfrewcenter.com

The Renfrew Center is an international organization dedicated to the better understanding and treatment of eating disorders. The website is packed with information.

www. paballet.org

The website of Pennsylvania Ballet. The dancers, their stories, the choreography, listings of performances, behind the scenes glimpses. Real dancers with real stories of performance at the highest level.

There are many, many helpful websites for all dancers, but I think the ones listed above are really great!

FOUR HELPFUL APPS FOR IPAD OR IPHONE

- Ballet Lite/Ballet Index: Terms defined. Helpful pronunciation guides.
- Virtual Trainer: Define your goals. Exercises for specific target areas.
- Ballet News: Brief notes on what's happening in the world of dance.
- GoodGuide: Featured in *The New York Times*. A guide to the actual environmental impact of certain products on the health of the world ecology as well as your own health.

THE NEW YORK TIMES

Excellent arts reporting with extensive dance coverage (and not only in the New York area); it helps you to become aware of dancers, dance companies and the larger dance world.

FIVE HELPFUL BOOKS

- Eric Franklin, *Dynamic Alignment through Imagery*. Champaign, IL (1996). If you do not read one word of this book, just looking through the illustrations will still be fascinating for you. This book, by a master teacher whose work has inspired many dancers and teachers, will change the way you think about your body and dance. Franklin has published a series of books on imagery for dance, fitness and good health. I think this book is a good place to start. Well worth the cost.

- Linda Hamilton, *The Dancer's Way: The New York City Ballet Guide to Mind, Body, and Nutrition*. NY: St. Martin's Press (2009). This excellent resource by dance psychologist Linda Hamilton is crammed with helpful tips on staying healthy while dancing. The book has particularly helpful sections on stress management and weight management. Dr. Hamilton is a columnist for *Dance Magazine* and a former dancer with the New York City Ballet. Dr. Hamilton has published several very helpful books regarding optimum health practices for the dancer and dance student.

- Justin Howse, *Dance Technique and Injury Prevention*, 3rd *Edition*. NY: Theatre Arts Books/Routledge (1988). Dr. Howse was one of the first physicians to seriously try to understand what was different about dance in terms of athletic injuries. His thoughtful analysis of the technique of various dance movements that might contribute to injury has been a model for medical researchers in dance medicine. The book includes many pictures relating to the exercises that dancers can do to help prevent injury.

- Ruth Solomon, John Solomon and Sandra Cerny Minton, eds., *Preventing Dance Injuries*, 2nd *Edition*. Champaign, IL: Human Kinetics (2005). Everything is in here. Everything. The editors have done an exhaustive survey of dance literature and compiled it all for you! Well worth a look as a place to start thinking about dancers' health.

Index

RC
1220
.D35
P48
2011